ASIAPAC PUBLICATION

Essence of Healthy Eating

Dietary Therapy in Traditional Chinese Medicine

By Cai Jingfeng

ASIAPAC • SINGAPORE

Publisher
ASIAPAC BOOKS PTE LTD
996 Bendemeer Road #06-09
Singapore 339944
Tel: (65) 6392 8455
Fax: (65) 6392 6455
Email: asiapacbooks@pacific.net.sg

Come visit us at our Internet home page
www.asiapacbooks.com

First published 1991 as *Eating Your Way to Health*

This Southeast Asian Edition
First published 1991 as *Nature's Way to Healthy Eating*

2nd edition (revised) October 2003
3rd edition July 2005

ISBN 981-229-324-8

Cover design by Chin Boon Leng
Printed in Singapore by Loi Printing Pte Ltd

Publisher's Note

Health is wealth, as the old adage goes. And the way to amass such wealth is to eat wisely, choosing the nourishing foods that nature offers so abundantly.

Dietary therapy is really the eating aspect in preventive health measures, which also embrace adequate rest, recreation and a healthy lifestyle. In the wake of SARS (Severe Acute Respiratory Syndrome), the basics of health maintenance is again emphasised — eating well to build a strong immunity against illnesses and diseases. The Chinese, with their long tradition of herbs and tonics, have handed down everyday knowledge of food therapy to promote health and longevity in an inexpensive way.

To make it easier for our readers to put this book into practice, we have appended a glossary of common medicinal foods in both English and Chinese. This book is highly accessible, and may be read alongside our publications on Chinese cuisine and traditional Chinese medicine.

To our readers: *bon appétit* and good health!

Related Titles (illustrated)
Essence of Traditional Chinese Medicine
Origins of Chinese Cuisine
Origins of Chinese Food Culture

About the Author

Cai Jingfeng was born in 1927 and graduated from the Hunan Medical College (Hunan-Yale Medical College) in 1954. He then studied traditional Chinese medicine for two and half years, and is now the head of the Second Department of the Institute of Chinese Medical History and Medical Literature under the Academy of Traditional Chinese Medicine. An associate professor in medical history, he specializes in both modern and traditional medicine, Chinese medical history and the medical history of minority nationalities.

He has published about one hundred academic papers, including "A History of Malaria in China", "A History of Infectious Hepatitis in China", "A History of Measles in China", "A Brief History of Anaesthesia in Traditional Chinese Medicine", "Li Shizhen's Scientific Achievements", and "The Origin and Evolution of the Theory of Channels and Collaterals".

Professor Cai is a member of the editorial board of the *Chinese Journal of Medicine, The Unabridged Dictionary of Traditional Chinese Medicine* and *The Concise Dictionary of Traditional Chinese Medicine*. He is an advisory editor of the *Journal of Traditional Chinese Medicine* (English edition) and *Medicine in Foreign Countries — Traditional Chinese Medicine* volume, and deputy editor-in-chief of the *Chinese Medicine Encyclopaedia* (volume on medical history), Traditional Chinese Medicine Biography Section. Recently, he has been elected a member of the standing committee of the Society of History of Medicine, Chinese Medical Association.

CONTENTS

I. WHAT IS DIETOTHERAPY?

I suppose many readers are annoyed by taking medicines when you get ill. Some such medicines are very peculiar, particularly those decoctions made from herbal compounds which are both bitter, hot, sour and puckery, and some of the tastes are so strange that one cannot tell what they are! However, for the sake of treatment, what else can one do but pinch his nose and swallow it down.

Things might be even worse when your sick child is not obedient. He might run off as soon as he sees the medicine. What then can you do? You have to seize him, constrain him to open his mouth, and pour the medicine down his throat by pinching his nostrils. Unfortunately, if the process is not properly handled, liquid may escape down the trachea causing even more complications.

How nice it would be if the decoction to be taken could be made of foodstuff or taste like food!

Dietotherapy refers to the treatment of disease by taking common foodstuffs, which, in China, are sometimes called by the name of medicinal foods. The intake of food is necessary for the maintenance of everyone's daily life and activity. Food contains the various nutrients which provide the energy supply for the body's growth and activities. The old Chinese saying that "Food is the No. 1 need for the people" reflects the utmost importance of food in daily life.

Note: Dietotherapy is also referred to as dietary therapy.

Nutrients are essential for people during illness to overcome pathogenic factors and repair tissue damage, and to resist and prevent diseases while in good health.

The art of dietotherapy roughly includes the following: Firstly, investigating the nature of food for preventing and treating diseases. In this sense, food itself is a remedy. For instance, in scurvy, a disease due to vitamin C deficiency, the eating of oranges, tangerines, or other fruits which are rich in vitamin C is helpful. Again, garlic behaves both as a food and as a remedy for bacillary dysentery. Secondly, investigating curative effects achieved by carefully selecting certain kinds of drug and adding them to food to complement each other. For instance, rice porridge is readily digested and nutritionally beneficial to patients. However, when radix discoreae, poria, or coix seeds are added, the porridge would have a strong anti-diarrhoea action by strengthening the spleen and improving digestion.

At present, the content of dietotherapy is being expanded. During the last few decades, cancer and cardiovascular diseases have replaced infectious diseases as the major enemy to human health. These two categories of disorders, especially cardio-vascular diseases, are closely tied to food habits. Coronary heart disease, the most common cardiovascular disease, results from high blood cholesterol which accumulates on the walls of the coronary vessels and leads to sclerosis. This process takes a long time to develop, say eight to ten years, or even as long as several decades. However, laboratory investigations reveal that signs of such pathologic change in the coronary vessels can begin to appear during a person's thirties or even earlier. This reminds us that, so long as we pay attention to and reasonably adjust our daily food and drink, the process of arteriosclerosis can be greatly postponed or even prevented. Therefore, it is advisable, for macrobiotic purposes, to start one's diet regimen as early as possible, preventing the onset of obesity or overweight.

Dietotherapy should include two further closely interwoven aspects, namely, the development of cooking technique to produce tasty foods, and the study of new foods that have therapeutic potential and their recipes.

Recently, the contents of traditional Chinese dietotherapy have been enriched by the further study of foods that are useful for preventing diseases and strengthening body resistance, cooking technique for dietotherapeutic purposes, and the combining or contradiction of foodstuffs.

Chinese dietotherapy, as a natural therapy, has also been welcomed in many other countries. Mr. Sasada, a Japanese scholar, assessed in his paper entitled "Research into Modern Classics on Diet", those works relevant to food from the period of the Song and Yuan dynasties onwards. In his opinion, ancient Chinese dietary study should embrace general works on food and drink, delicacies of all sorts and also ordinary foods eaten by the common people. He concluded that such works amounted to as many as 38 in the Song-Yuan dynasties, 41 in the Ming Dynasty, and 40 in the Qing Dynasty.

All the above facts show that Chinese dietotherapy is a special branch of science with a wide and unique content.

II. CHINA'S AGE-OLD DIETOTHERAPY

As everyone knows, living organisms require nutrients taken in from outside the body for the maintenance of life. Animals, especially the higher animals, require more complex nutrients supplied by a great variety of foods.

The earliest Homo Sapiens had to find food. During this search, they gradually learned how to select edible foods avoiding poisonous ones, a process which may be viewed, in the broadest sense, as the earliest dietotherapy. Hence, the old Chinese saying: "Shen Nong tried everything, tasting the plants and sampling the waters in order to tell his people what to eat and what to avoid. Indeed, out of every hundred, he found seventy poisonous plants."* This vividly depicts primitive dietotherapy and the process of finding edible foods.

The life of primitive man was a savage one. At that time, "Man took wild fruits, clams, and other rank and foul foods harmful to the digestive tract, causing many diseases among the people."** After the use of fire was mastered, however, raw foods were eaten cooked. Cooked food is not only tasty, but also greatly lessens the chance of contracting diseases, especially those through the

---

*Chapter on Self-discipline, *Book of Prince Huai Nan*, by Liu An (179 BC-122 BC) of the Western Han Dynasty.

**Chapter on Five Worms, *Book of Han Fei*, by Han Fei (280 BC-233 BC) of the Warring States Period.

digestive tract. Cooked food strengthens the body's resistance to disease, since the nutrients in the food, especially the proteins, are more readily digested and absorbed. What is more, the pathogenic microbes contaminating food are mostly destroyed on cooking, thus greatly reducing the chance of illness. This is reflected in the old saying that "Sui Ren (fire man) invented fire by drilling wood and instructed the people to take cooked food to prevent digestive diseases".* Obviously, Shen Nong and Sui Ren are both legendary figures. The discovery and development of agriculture and the application of fire cannot be attributed to any one individual, being, of course, the result of the accumulated experiences of primitive man over the ages. However, the legend does reflect, more or less, the actual process of the human experience of strengthening body resistance and preventing disease through food processing and cooking.

It is, of course, a very long process from avoiding disease by selecting foods to consciously utilizing foods for the treatment and preventing of diseases.

In the *Inner Classic of the Yellow Emperor*,** China's earliest extant theoretical medical text, the foundations of a etiology, pathology, pathogenesis, treatment and prevention are laid down, as is the theoretical basis for dietotherapy. This work points out that irregular eating and drinking can cause disease, and that greasy and rich diets are not readily digestible, while over-burdening the gastro-intestinal tract by too much eating would result in disease. In light of this, the classic laid down a series of principles and methods for treating and pre-

---

**Book of Rites*, said to be written by the Duke of Zhou, a politician of the 11th century BC and revised by Confucius (551 BC-479 BC).

**This Classic was first compiled between the 4th and 1st centuries BC, and is now composed of two books, *Plain Questions* and *The Miraculous Pivot*.

venting diseases with dietotherapy, saying that, "When using medicines of drastic toxicity for treatment, application should be interrupted when the illness is about 60% ameliorated or cured; for medicines of moderate toxicity, when 70% cured; for medicines with slight toxicity, when 80% cured; for non-toxic medicines, when 90% cured. The remaining illness should be treated by following a proper diet, for otherwise an excessive use of medicines will bring harmful results." This means that medicines which are to a greater or lesser degree toxic to the body should be applied with care, interrupted in time, and then supplanted by dietotherapy. In other words, proper food and drink form the basis for the treatment of illness. *Plain Questions* of the *Inner Classic* also points out "... grains for growth, fruits for assistance, meat for nutrition and vegetables for supplement". It is quite clear that ancient Chinese physicians paid great attention to the combining of all kinds of food so as to maintain normal health and support body resistance, as well as for conquering pathogens when ill. For instance, some of the few prescriptions which appear in the *Inner Classic* are actually common dietotherapeutic ones.

On this theoretical basis, dietotherapy developed further in the Han Dynasty (206 BC-AD 220). The earliest Chinese monograph of materia medica still extant, *Shen Nong's Classic of Herbology*, compiled during this period, is exclusively concerned with the nature, flavour, action and growing place of medical substances. It lists some 365 kinds divided into three categories, namely superior, intermediate and inferior, including 67 kinds of animal and 252 herbal substances. Among them, some are foods that can be administered over a long period to benefit the body, such as the Chinese date, Chinese yam, coix seed, etc. It also states that sargassum is good for thyroid disease. Others, like sesame, grape, honey, walnut, longan, and lily bulb, are all common fruits and foods. This clearly illustrates that there was a stage when the distinction between medicines and foods blurred.

The distinguished physician of the Eastern Han Dynasty (25-220), Zhang Zhongjing, paid great attention to dietotherapy in his *Synopsis of the Golden Chamber*, saying that "... food and drink are beneficial to health, but only when taken appropriately both as to quality and quantity; otherwise, they can become detrimental. Moreover, for sick persons, suitable food will be beneficial to the recovery from illness, while unsuitable food aggravates the condition". He then goes on to mention several dozen pairs of contradictory foods, for example, crab and persimmon, macrostem onion and beef, etc. In another of his works, *The Treatise on Febrile Diseases*, there are many instances in which he applies dietotherapy. The first prescription in the book called the Decoction of Cinnamon Twigs contains cinnamon twigs, radix paeonial alba (white peony root), zingiberis (fresh ginger), radix glycy rrhiza (liquorice root) and fructus ziziphi jujubae (Chinese dates). Three of these five ingredients are both a food or flavouring and a medicine. When applying this decoction, not only the decoction is taken, a bowl of warm rice porridge is also advisable to promote the blood and vital energy circulation so as to strengthen the action of the decoction, and to induce a slight sweat helping expel pathogen. Prescriptions such as the Pig Skin Decoction, Lily Bulb with Egg Decoction and Radix Angelica, Ginger and Mutton Decoction in *The Treatise on Febrile Diseases* are all typical dietotherapeutic prescriptions. This last prescription is still applied clinically,being a tonic commonly given to women resting after child-birth, especially during the autumn and winter months.

The Sui (581-618) and Tang (618-907) dynasties saw

further understanding of dietotherapy. Sun Simiao (581-673) has in his masterpiece, *Thousand Gold Remedies for Emergencies*, a chapter devoted exclusively to dietotherapy, saying that "doctors should first understand the pathogenesis of the disease, and then treat it with diet. Drugs should only be used if diet fails". This is a very scientific attitude towards the treatment of disease. For any kind of medicine is "toxic", in the medical sense, to the pathogens that cause disease, and it is by this "toxicity" that medicines cure disease, attacking the pathogens and restoring the body's functions. However, this toxicity may also cause a certain degree of damage to the host tissue. That is why ancient physicians called medicines "toxic" substances. However, dietotherapy does not have such shortcomings. It cures disease by adjusting body functions and strengthening resistance through nutritional supplements. That is why dietotherapy was so emphasized, especially for consumptive disease, in this period. Sun Simiao also pointed out that only those adept in dietotherapy could be called superb or excellent physicians. His dietotherapy chapter, considered to be the first monograph of its kind in Chinese medical history, mentions many dieto-prescriptions, including animal liver for night-blindness, sargassum for lymphadenitis, chaff coix seed and red bean for beriberi, etc.

Another monograph on dietotherapy from the Tang Dynasty, *Mastery of Dietotherapy* by Zan Yin, embraces thirteen sections about dietotherapy for internal medicine, gynaecological and paediatrical diseases, with a total of some two hundred prescriptions. Even apoplexy and cold colic of the heart and abdomen are included. Meng Shen, one of Sun Simiao's disciples, wrote *Herbs for Dietotherapy*, later revised by his disciple Zhang Ding into a 3-volume monograph with 227 sections including 241 medicinal foods. Though the original was lost, a remnant of over twenty sections was discovered in the Dunhuang Grottoes in 1907 and is now in the British Museum.

Food prohibition is another important part of dietotherapy. Its contents are rather meticulous, for instance, raw, cold, mucilaginous, spicy meat or fish foods should be especially avoided in certain diseases. Breaking of these prohibitions would result in the worsening of disease or lead to a relapse, what is called a "food relapse". For instance, in traditional Chinese medicine, jaundice is believed to be the result of evil dampness and heat accumulated in the spleen-stomach, hence mucilaginous food and foods of a hot and dry nature are to be avoided; crab meat, on the other hand, is not appropriate for asthmatic patients; alcohol is prohibited for apopletics, etc. Contradiction was an important issue at this period. It is mentioned in Chao Yuanfang's *General Treatise on the Etiology and Symptomology of Disease* that for febrile diseases, "when the disease is newly abated, the digestive system is very weak and the patient's resistance has not yet completely recovered, any pork, intestines, fish, bloody or greasy food, if taken, will result in incurable consequences. Also, mucilaginous grains, fish, date and other foods difficult to digest can result in severe pyretic relapse."

The Song Dynasty (960-1279) also saw great attention paid to dietotherapy. There are chapters relating to dietotherapy in all three medical books compiled by the Song imperial court, namely *The Peaceful Holy Benevolent Prescription*, *Prescriptions of the Bureau of People's Welfare Pharmacies*, and *General Collection for Holy Relief*. In the first work, for instance, dietotherapeutic prescriptions are divided into 29 categories, in 320 prescriptions, among which, milk to treat diabetes, carp porridge and black bean syrup to treat edema, apricot-nut and wild jujuba seed porridge to treat senile insommia, palpitations and night sweating, are convenient and effective dietotherapeutic prescriptions.

Another monograph of the same period, *The New Book for Providing for Parental Longevity*, recommends "fewer greasy foods for benefiting the blood and energy", and "optimal diets for cultivating the digestive functions" for the elderly. It also recommends well-cooked and warm foods for the elderly, and few hot and dry natured food for women, who should have more plain and tonic foods.

Being both simple and effective for treatment and prevention, dietotherapy was very common in the Song Dynasty. In Wu Zhimu's *A Record of Dreams in the Capital Lin'an* is depicted the lively and vivid society of the capital Lin'an (present-day Hangzhou). Deep into the night the market would gradually calm down and just before dawn, vendors of medicinal porridge would already be out and about.

The Jin (1115-1234) and Yuan (1206-1368) dynasties saw continued development in the art of dietotherapy. The four great physicians of this period, Liu Wansu (1120-1200), Zhang Zihe (1156-1228), Li Dongyuan (1180-1251) and Zhu Danxi (1281-1358) devoted some space to dietotherapy in their works. For example, Zhang Zihe explicitly points out that "those deficient in blood and semen should build themselves up with food", while dietotherapy was even more essential to the Benefiting School of Zhu Danxi. Most of his prescriptions for tonification include animal fats and proteins. One of his tonic pills was actually composed of pig's brain and spinal cord.

Viewing diet from a nutritional point of view was a special content of dietotherapy in this period. *The Essential of Foods*, written by a Mongolian, Hu Sihui, is the earliest monograph on nutrition. The author stressed not only the treatment of disease by food but also the improving of body resistance through nutrition. He emphasized that the elderly should take more nutritional foods, such as mutton, porridge, pig's liver, eggs, milk, etc. On the basis of some 60 years of experience the author recorded 214 kinds of food, of which 31 are made from grain, 31 animal, 17 fowl, 22 fish, 89 fruit, and 46 vegetable, including a further 28 condiments, some of them characterized by particular national features, such as Mongolian or Uygur milk products. Another important work of the same period, *The Daily Herbology*, records 540 kinds of medicine divided into eight categories, namely rice, grain, vegetable, fruit, fowl, beast, fish and worm.

Quite a number of dietotherapy works appeared in the Ming (1368-1644) and Qing (1644-1911) dynasties. Some of them dealt with the nutritional value of food; others discussed the therapeutic nature of food, classifying foods on the basis of their therapeutic action. The distinguished naturalist Li Shizhen (1518-1593) classed water as the first medicine in his masterpiece, *Encyclopaedia of Materia Medica*, saying that "Water is the origin of all things on the globe — drink comes from water, while food comes from earth. Food and drink are of vital importance to human life". This demonstrates his awareness of the importance of water as food. He also mentions some fifty kinds of porridge. Zhu Shu's *Herbs for Famine Relief* is devoted exclusively to the wild plants which can serve as food during famine and disaster, thus greatly expanding the range of human food and mastering another development in dietotherapy. In addition, Gao Lian's *Eight Treatises for Preserving Longevity* included thirty-two dietotherapeutic prescriptions and thirty-five medicinal porridges.

In this period, monographs on medicinal porridge began to appear, most notably, Huang Boxiong's *Mirror of Herbology for Dietotherapy* which mentions one hundred kinds of medicinal porridge, another unique characteristic of traditional Chinese dietotherapy.

To sum up, dietotherapy is an integral part of traditional Chinese medicine which embraces a wide variety of contents of great value to mankind. It has made great contributions to human health and will, undoubtedly, continue to do so.

III. THE NATURE AND FLAVOUR OF FOOD

The study of dietotherapy has not only a theoretical foundation, but is also of active, practical significance. When a person falls ill, treatment is required. Except for some individual ailments (such as diabetes), a person suffering from illness always has a bad appetite, and is averse to the taking of food and drink, to say nothing of medicines. This is an impediment to the healing process and physical recovery. The chief good of traditional dietotherapy is, by making use of the therapeutic nature of the foods themselves (including some medicinal foods and a few straight medicines), by the careful manipulation and cooking of the food, and by the appropriate compounding of food and a small amount of medicine, to stimulate the appetite of the patient so as to aid the cure of disease.

A. The Common Origins of Medicine and Food

There is an old saying that "Traditional medicine and food share a common origin". In other words, medicine and food have the same origin but different usages. In remote prehistory, there must have been a period when medicine and food were both eaten indiscriminately without any distinct demarcation. This is simply due to the fact that primitive man could not yet tell medicine from food. It was not until a long time later that people began to differentiate a few substances with clear therapeutic action from common foods.

Legend has it that around the 11th century BC, King Tang of the Shang Dynasty had an excellent chief, named Yi Yin, who also used to cook soups for his king when he was ill. Having drunk a few bowls of the soup, the king would then recover. Hence, Yi Yin is reputed to be the inventor of decoctions. Whatever the real story, this legend reflects that the soups and the decoctions share a common origin. This common origin of food and medicine is also reflected in the position of wine. Wine has been very popular since ancient times. However, it also became of great importance in medicine, so much that both the Chinese characters for "medicine" (醫) and "wine" (酒) have the same component " 酉 " as their radicals.

Dietotherapy is based, then, on this common origin of medicine and food. In traditional Chinese medicine, many common foods serve as medicines and many specific medicines are also commonly used foodstuffs. Among others, Chinese date, ginger, cinnamon, Chinese prickly ash, Chinese onion, garlic, Chinese yam, liquor, vinegar, eggs, sesame, mung bean, apricot kernal and rice are the most common.

In brief, there are plenty of natural products that possess such a dual property, and it is hard to say whether they are foodstuff or medicine. Habitually, we call those which are taken daily or quite often and can be consumed over a long period of time without detrimental effect foodstuffs, whereas those which are not palatable, not in daily use and produce a distinct physiological reaction are called medicines or drugs.

Moreover, it is customary to get medicines from a drug store or dispensary and foodstuffs from a grocery. This phenomenon is actually the result of social progress and the division of social work. As bestowed by nature, medicines are not easy to distinguish from foods, and strictly speaking, most medicines were isolated from foodstuffs. A certain substance which revealed a marked reaction when swallowed and could not be taken for a long course nor repeatedly was isolated from ordinary foodstuffs and treated as "medicine". When the body is discomforted to such an extent that it becomes necessary to apply such "food" capable of producing dramatic action to cure that discomfort, this is treatment with "medicine". Gradually, medicines were isolated from the family of food. However, foodstuffs such as cinnamon, Chinese date, pepper, Chinese prickly ash, lotus root, pumpkin seed, walnut, longan, crystal sugar, hawthorn, seed of Job's tear and many other herbs, spices and other natural products can be bought from a herbalist's or a grocery shop and are used both for daily cooking and as medicine.

In order to maintain normal daily activity, the body needs energy, which is supplied by food and drink. When the body wants for energy, discomfort or abnormal sensations are felt. For instance, when one feels hungry, if food is not supplied in time, one may experience dizziness, palpitations, perspiration, and weakness. This is a temporary reaction called hypoglycemia and it can be immediately set right if food is supplied in time. Probably everyone has experienced this himself at some time or another. However, this condition is not generally viewed as pathological, since it is a kind of physiological reaction. It can thus be seen that the two states are relative rather than absolute, with no sharp demarcation between, just as in the case of food and medicine. Without food, the normal physiological state will change into a pathological one, while improper food supply, either excessive or deficient, especially to those with special needs such as the elderly and pregnant women, would result in a breakdown of physical health.

These two concepts, the relative relationship between the pathological and normal condition and the common origins of food and medicine, provide the foundation and starting point for dietotherapy in traditional Chinese medicine.

B. The Nature and Flavour of Food

Traditional Chinese medicine lays great stress on the nature and flavour of materia medica. There are four natures: cold, hot, warm, and cool; and five flavours: salty, sour, sweet, bitter and pungent. Since in traditional Chinese medicine the application of antagonistic therapy is emphasized by using medicine with the opposite nature and flavour to that of the illness, so it is of great significance to explore and master the characteristics of medicines in order to achieve "neutralization," i.e., a harmonized state of the body.

In traditional Chinese medicine, it is held that the human body is healthy when it is in a harmonious state. A preponderance of any condition would result in disease. For instance,disease may manifest itself as cold or hot, deficient or excessive in nature. Acute diseases manifesting high fever, thirst, headaches, deep-coloured urine, etc., are often said to be of a hot and excessive nature, while chronic diseases of long duration, with hypo functions and bad circulation manifesting as cold extremities, chilliness, emaciation, short breath, etc., are said to be cold and deficient in nature. For hot diseases of a severe case, cold remedies should be used, while for mild cases, cool remedies should be applied. In contrast, for those cold diseases of a severe case, hot remedies are indicated, while warm medicines are prescribed for mild diseases of a cold nature.

It goes without saying that, since dietotherapy is a kind of treatment, it should obey the same principles as medicinal therapy in order to overcome the preponderance of a condition causing disorder. In other words, similar attention should be paid to the nature and flavour of food and drink. For instance, among common foods, coriander is warm, pepper is hot, balsam pear is cold and bean curd is cool in nature. Moreover,baked, fried and broiled foods are all hot and dry in nature, while greasy and mucilaginous foods tend to transform, once eaten, into heat or evil-hot dampness. Vegetables and fruits, with few exceptions, are cool and sour. Naturally, one must pay attention to the natures of these foods so as to achieve good results with treatment. An illness of a hot nature will be worsened by taking mutton, dog's meat, chicken, pepper, cinnamon, dried ginger, longan or lichee which are all of a warm or hot nature. Similarly, those suffering from diseases of a cold nature should avoid taking foods such as sugar cane, water chestnut, water melon, balsam pear, etc. which are believed to be cold or cool in nature.

Regarding the five flavours, i.e., salty, sour, sweet, bitter and pungent, each has its own pharmacological action which has been determined by theory and through long experience and practice in daily life. Accordingly, traditional Chinese medicine theory claims that salty medicines are good at softening lumps; pungent medicines for dispersing the vital energy throughout the body, which is helpful for eliminating evil pathogens, and so are commonly applied for common cold and flu; sweet medicines, for deficient diseases, although excess sweat is harmful to the appetite; sour medicines for astringent action, treating loss of body fluid, such as in diarrhoea or excess sweating, and for activating blood circulation; bitter medicines for antipyretic use, elimination of dampness and stimulating the appetite.

Actions from the five flavours of foods are basically the same as those from medicines. Bitter foods are antipyretic, such as fermented soya bean, balsam pear, animal bile, etc; sweet foods are fluid secretion promoting, Yin nourishing and also antipyretic, such as lotus root, potato, radix rehmanial, radix dioscoreal (Chinese yam), radix polygonati (sealwort), semen coicis (coix seed), sweet potato, sugar cane and water-melon, most starch-rich foods being in this class. Sour foods are astringent, blood activating and stagnation eliminating, such as hawthorn, wild jujube, vinegar, apricot, tomato and the like. Pungent foods are capable of dispersing evil cold and wind, such as Chinese onion, ginger, prickly ash peel, mustard and chilli, and these are commonly applied for the initial stage of common cold, when the invading evil cold and wind still remain in the superficial part of the body. Salty food refers to innate salty foods rather than those processed with salt, for instance, foods from the sea such as seaweed and kelp are innately salty foods, and are capable of softening lumps, such as goitres, tuberculous lymph glands, etc.

In order to achieve a satisfactory therapeutic result, it is essential to take the nature and flavour of foodstuffs into overall account. In medicinal therapy, drugs of a hot nature, like ephedra and cinnamon twigs, are applied in severe cold diseases, while for mildly cold ailments, only honeysuckle flower and forsythia fruit are applied. These rules are similarly applicable in dietotherapy, and the action of the food whether mild or drastic, should be discriminated. For instance, onions and ginger are strongly hot, while raw brown sugar, and turnip are warm. They should be chosen for treatment according to the severity of the ailment. However, most foods always possess two or even more kinds of flavour, some being both sour and sweet, others both pungent and bitter, while their nature may be rather simple, either hot or cold, warm or cool. Hence, one must have a thorough understanding of their natures and flavours in order to put them to effective use and cure the disease.

As a rule, severe and acute diseases should be treated by medicines or a combination of medicines with dietotherapy, while for chronic ailments, dietotherapy is highly recommended. Medicines, no matter how simple their action, often produce certain unexpected and disadvantageous side effects. With dietotherapy such shortcomings can be avoided even over a long period of therapy.

C. The Compounding and Cooking of Medicinal Food

The compounding of a medicinal diet is very important, since inappropriate compounding would result in ineffectiveness or even produce harmful effects on the patient. For instance, persimmon ripens in autumn and dried persimmon porridge is a food traditionally eaten at this time by the elderly to strengthen the spleen and benefit the lungs. However, if crabs, which are also most commonly available in autumn, are eaten at the same time as persimmons, this will cause harm to patients by weakening digestive functions. This is due to the coagulation of the protein in the crabmeat through reaction with tannic acid from the persimmon, sometimes even causing gastric stones, making digestion difficult. This phenomenon was mentioned as early as in Zhang Zhongjing's *Synopsis of the Golden Chamber*, in which he points out many such food prohibitions, such as asthma patients eating too much gingko, or those with chronic diarrhoea, too much dried longan or Chinese date. Satisfactory results can only be obtained when the correct dose and compounding are combined, otherwise it may be harmful.

China is well known for her cookery. While most of the cooking techniques used in dietotherapy are the same as those of ordinary cookery, dietotherapy does, however, have some particular characteristics.

Chinese cookery includes many different methods, such as boiling, frying, baking, broiling, steaming, stir-frying, stir-frying with starch, stir-frying with soybeans, stewing, braising, sauté, quick-frying, and so on. The aim of these different techniques, however diversified, is to arouse and improve the appetite of the consumer, through the attractive colour, smell and taste of the food. Medicinal food should be of harmonious and pleasing appearance, fragrance appealing, to arouse the patient's appetite. The demands for dietotherapeutic cookery are technically higher than for ordinary cookery. Since most patients lose their appetite, badly cooked food would further depress the patient's appetite, thus forming a vicious cycle harmful to convalescence. As most medicines have a peculiar or unpleasant smell, it goes without saying that medicinal food needs to be skilfully cooked to give it a pleasant and enticing aroma. A good medicinal chef can cook delicious medicinal dishes and foods so that the patient does not realize that medicine is being taken. In so doing, disease is cured unconsciously simply by eating. Besides its attractive appearance medicinal food should also be readily digestable. Generally, such food should be light, easily digested and not greasy. High fatty and greasy foods are not readily digested and are appetite depressing, and so will not have the desired effect.

D. Varieties of Medicinal Food

There are many varieties of medicinal food. The following are the most common:

1. Porridge

This is a common form of medicinal food made of rice. The rice is first boiled at a high heat for a few minutes and then at a gentle heat until it becomes mucilaginous. Obviously, the right amount of water should be used. Too much water would make the porridge too thin, which is not effective, whereas too little water would make it too concentrated or make it into steamed rice, even perhaps burning it, which is clearly no good. In traditional Chinese medicine, non-glutinous rice is preferred to other grains. When suitably cooked, rice porridge provides sufficient energy and protects the functions of the spleen and stomach. It is believed in traditional Chinese medicine that when the vital energy of the stomach is "depleted", the disease will be incurable, and that is why rice porridge is considered to be the most fundamental of dietotherapeutic foods.

Millet, wheat and maize can also be used to make porridge; however, they are inferior to rice porridge. Glutinous rice is difficult to digest and hence is not so suitable to make porridge.

For medicinal porridge, the medicine can be either pulverized and added directly to the porridge for cooking, or prepared as a decoction in advance and then added.

2. Thick soup

Generally prepared from meat, fish or eggs. These soups are a medical treatment in themselves. For instance, carp soup and pig's liver soup are all highly nutritious and good for deficiency ailments. Mild medicines can also be added, such as powdered ginger, white of Chinese onion, pepper, *Lycium chinensis* or fermented soy beans, some of which may increase nourishment value; some may improve eyesight; and some may serve as mild diaphretics to relieve the exterior symptom complex. Medicines of a strong nature can also be added, either prepared in advance and then added or cooked at the same time. In some provinces in south China like Fujian and Guangdong, it is customary to stew chicken, duck, soft-shelled tortoise, pig's heart, pig's liver or pork with radix cengelica, rhizoma ligusticum wallichii, radix, astragalus membraraceus, *Lycium chinensis*, etc. These medicines add both taste, nourishment and curative effect. Synergitic efficacy results in such cases by the reciprocal action between the soup and medicine complementing each other.

3. Drink

This is another common form of dietotherapy. Drink, different from thick soup, which is made from foods with rather high protein and fat ingredients, is mostly made from light foods of thin flavour infused in boiling water. Tea-like infusions are most common. Such drinks are mostly made of flowers, leaves or fruits, such as chrysanthemum tea, hawthorn juice or made of ophiopogon japonicus. In traditional Chinese medicine, chrysanthemum and mulberry tea is the most common medicinal drink. By drink, it means a liquid which is to be sipped little by little from time to time. Also common are honey drink, sweet black tea, and a drink made from sterculia scaphigera.

4. Staple food

Staple food here refers to, aside from the aforementioned porridge, foods made of rice, flour and other grains, sometimes with medicinal herbs added. However, it is essential that his staple medicinal food should have no special taste or smell, or at least, very little. For instance, a kind of cake eaten by people in China made of poris coces pulverized with rice powder, cane sugar and then steamed, is such a staple medicinal food without any special medicinal smell, and is universally accepted, even by children. This medicinal staple food is beneficial to the spleen, i.e. helpful to digestion and absorption.

Besides cakes, staple food can be also prepared for medicinal use in the form of pancakes, steamed cakes, steamed stuffed buns (either sweet or salty), steamed twisted rolls, sweet cakes, dumplings or steamed rice. Generally speaking, all daily forms of staple food can be prepared for medicinal purposes.

5. Dishes

To the Chinese, dishes are served as non-staple food. Though there are a great variety of cooking methods for medicinal food, since dietotherapy is applied chiefly in chronic diseases it mainly uses those methods of preparing food at a low heat over a rather long period, such as steaming, boiling, cooking with soy sauce and braising, during which the nutrients tend to be dissolved in the soup and are easily digested, this being more suitable for the patient. Those methods, such as frying, baking, and broiling, believed to be hot in nature, are less applied for medicinal use. Whatever kind of cooking technique one adopts, the flavour, form, colour and aroma must be considered so as to arouse the patient's appetite.

6. Liquor

Liquor is a common beverage which can be applied for medicinal purposes and is another important form of dietotherapy. Liquor contains alcohol which is an excellent solvent and can dissolve more active constituents than other methods of cooking or decocting. Moreover, liquor lends its own action to bring the medicine's therapeutic potential into full play, stimulating or improving blood circulation to acquire special effect. Liquors containing sugar or residue (distillers grain) are called *li* or *liao* respectively, and both are of therapeutic significance. Preparation of medicinal liquor is simple, involving the immersion of segments or slices of the raw medicine into the liquor for a long period, or by putting both liquor and medicine into a pot, then heated by immersing in hot water.

7. Decoction

This traditional therapeutic method is probably the most widely used of all in China, possessing the advantages of being easily digested, easily handled and of reliable effect. In general, it is prepared by putting the raw medicines into water and then boiling, first with a strong heat and then with a low heat to keep it simmering in order to dissolve the active constituents. This decoction is then filtered and the residue discarded. The decoction is now ready for administration. Sometimes the residue is also eaten, since not all the active constituents are extracted out into the decoction. However, bitter and puckery residues are, as a rule, discarded. Decoctions can also be prepared by placing the container in a steamer or water bath, which is a method used for valuable medicines such as ginseng, tremella, etc.

8. Juice

Juices are mostly prepared from fruits or the roots, stem tubers, leaves or fruits of vegetables. Being mostly cold in nature, they are commonly applied for replenishing body fluid. For the elderly, weak, and especially those patients convalescing after a high fever, it is a useful form of nourishment. The juice is prepared by wrapping the pieces of fresh fruit or vegetable in a gauze and then pressing them, or simply by using a press. It is advisable to drink the juice while fresh, especially during the summer, otherwise being sure to keep it in the refrigerator. The juice should not be boiled, or its vitamin C content will be destroyed.

9. Honey paste

Also known as nourishing paste due to its tonic actions. It is prepared by mildly heating the juice extracted from fresh fruit, plants or vegetables until most of the water is evaporated, leaving a rather sticky paste into which honey is then added. Honey paste is both tasty and nourishing, and is suitable for all patients of different ages. It is usually kept in a large jar, and one teaspoonful is administered either diluted with water or swallowed directly.

10. Preserved fruits or sweets

Sugar, either white or brown, is used as a base. It is mixed with water and gently heated until very sticky, so that when cooled it will become hard. When heating, medicine in powdered or liquid form is poured in, thus forming medicinal sweets. Preserved fruits are usually made by immersing fruits or some medicinal materials in honey or cane sugar for a considerable period of time.

IV. ADMINISTERING MEDICINAL FOOD ON THE BASIS OF SYNDROME DIFFERENTIATION

Treating diseases according to syndrome differentiation is one of the most fundamental and unique aspects of traditional Chinese medicine. It involves the overall consideration of all the factors involved relevant to the patient's condition, including the symptoms, signs, and state of the disease itself, and the patient's age, sex, constitution, as well as climatic and geographic conditions and so on. Therefore, treatments are not mechanical or dogmatic, but rather adaptable and flexible. Dietotherapy is based on these same principles. This is what we call administering dietotherapy on the basis of syndrome differentiation.

A. Administering Dietotherapy in Accordance with Different Individuals, Places and Seasons

The constitution of each individual varies just as facial features do. Likewise, each individual has his own preference for and reaction to different foods. For instance, some people like strong-smelling preserved bean curd, while others detest it; milk is a common drink to some, while to others it may cause diarrhoea; cucumber is a very common food to most of us; however, it may cause allergic reactions to some individuals, producing abdominal pain, diarrhoea, vomiting or fever.

An individual's constitution may be classed as cold, hot, deficient or excessive. Generally speaking, an individual of deficient constitution should take more nutritious food, while this is not necessary for those individuals of an excessive constitution. Strangely enough, some deficient individuals simply cannot accept nourishing foods, which only cause them discomfort, and they can only take common or plain foods. For those with a hot constitution, hot and dried foods made by frying,baking or roasting should be avoided. Certain individuals can stand up to one pound of longan or lichi without any reaction, while others suffer from epistaxis (nose bleeds) after having eaten only ten pieces. A fat person is said to have a high phlegm and wet constitution and should take more foods which are plain and easily digested, whereas thin persons are said to be deficient and should take more nourishing and fluid promoting foods. In brief, dietotherapy quite obviously should be administered according to the needs and constitutions of different individuals and should never be applied indiscriminately.

Seasonal changes are another important factor in the application of dietotherapy. Medicinal food should vary according to the different seasons. For instance, during the hot summer months it is not feasible to prescribe a diet of a dry, hot or greasy nature; instead, plain, cool and non-greasy foods are preferable. On cold winter days, however, nourishing paste or even a little greasy food is recommended. According to the traditional view, even the food eaten at specific times within a single day should vary. It is advisable to take easily digested, non-greasy food for breakfast, and greasy and nourishing food for lunch. It is highly recommended not to take greasy food or food difficult to digest at supper and after an early supper, eating no more prior to going to bed.

Geographical conditions are also important. For instance, China is a vast country and when the northern part is still deep frozen, the southern part is already blooming into colour. For northern inhabitants, nourishing pastes or slightly greasy foods, even foods of a hot nature, are permissible, while for southerners, foods of a cold nature and those easily digested, rather than greasy foods, are preferred. Moreover, inhabitants in different parts of the country have widely differing habits regarding food and drink. Some prefer pungent and spicy foods; others prefer sour, sweet or salty diets. It all depends on the climatic and geographical conditions which lead to the development of habits and customs over many generations. Investigations should be made at the time the therapy is carried out, so as to avoid incompatibility and troubles due to neglect of differences in climate, habits or personal physical constitutions.

B. The Main Purpose of Dietotherapy — Nourishing

During illness, the body requires an increase in nutrients and energy to combat the pathogens and aid the recovery of normal functioning. However, the relevant nerve centres are inhibited and digestive functions greatly reduced, the sick body refusing to take the extra food required for raising resistance. The main task of dietotherapy is to try to resolve this contradiction, not only providing medicinal treatment, but also improving the patient's appetite so that the additional nourishment provided can be assimilated.

Of course, dietotherapy is not only concerned with treatment. Equally important is prevention of disease. In the *Inner Classic of the Yellow Emperor*, it is said that a "superior physician" is one who treats before illness arises. To administer medicines after the disease has already developed could be likened to digging a well after one feels thirsty, and forging weapons after one has already engaged in battle. The positive significance of Chinese dietotherapy lies in its prevention rather than in its treatment; treating when there is disease and preventing before disease actually happens. This point was clearly recognized in early traditional Chinese medicine; for instance, in the Eastern Capital (now Kaifeng, Henan Province) of the Song Dynasty, on the 8th of the twelfth month (lunar calendar), all Buddhist temples had an "assembly for bathing the Buddha" during which "porridge of seven valuables and five flavours" was distributed which was believed to "expel noxious cold and eliminate diseases."

Dietotherapy is also applied according to the stage of the illness; for instance, when an acute or febrile disease is in its ascending or peak stage, greasy and nourishing food should be avoided, as this may further stimulate the disease.

In general, dietotherapy is mostly administered in cases of chronic disease, where the patient is usually of a deficient type. Traditional Chinese medicine emphasizes "assisting the patient's resistance to overcome the pathogenic factors". In this sense, benefiting or nourishing is important for supplementing the patient with nutrition and balancing the Yin-Yang principles. This issue is especially important for the elderly whose body functions are degenerating, and for women who, due to physiological characteristics, are liable to be insufficient both in blood and in energy. All such people are most benefited by nourishing diets. If an illness is in its acute stage then it is termed "excess" in traditional Chinese medicine and nourishing therapy should not be administered. Only once the pathogens have been expelled can benefiting therapy be applied.

The methods of benefiting or nourishing vary from plain nourishing to mild, warm and tonic nourishing. For instance, during the recovery stage of acute febrile diseases only a plain benefiting diet such as rice porridge should be administered.

C. Some Special Types of Medicinal Diet

1. For children

There is a great scope for the development of medicinal diets for children. As a rule, children are averse to swallowing medicines. Satisfactory therapeutic results can be obtained, though, if we take full advantage of dietotherapy.

Children readily accept such forms of dietotherapy as honey-preserved fruits, sweets, or porridges; however, they are susceptible to acute diseases, often with an overwhelming onset and of short duration, limiting the possible application of dietotherapy. Medicinal diets are mostly appropriate for children with chronic diseases. The most common of these is dyspepsia (bad digestion) which is caused by the over-eating of meat, greasy and other not easily digested foods, causing overwork on the stomach and intestines. Hawthorn and the like are the best foods for this kind of ailment. It may be prepared as hawthorn cake, preserved hawthorn in honey, hawthorn jelly, etc. Moreover, milk, yoghurt and all kinds of porridge which are beneficial to digestion are mostly favoured by children.

In brief, medicinal diets for children should be both easily digestible and tasty, and can be administered for a long period without any side-effects. Combining chiropractic with dietotherapy will yield even better results.

2. For women

After puberty, females experience a series of physiological processes, including menstruation, pregnancy, delivery and lactation. As a result, women need to consume more nutrients and energy than males of the same age.

During menstruation a fair amount of blood may be lost, and if the nutrients such as inorganic iron and protein for synthesizing haemoglobin are not supplemented there is the eventual possibility of contracting anaemia. Of course, such anaemia can readily be cured by administering mineral iron preparations, such as ferrous sulfate. However, since the latter is a kind of chemical drug, it may cause side-effects, such as abdominal discomfort or even pains. If iron-rich foods such as animal liver, eggs or even potherb mustard are supplied, such unexpected side-effects can be easily avoided.

During pregnancy, the mother-to-be needs exceptional amounts of calcium, phosphorus, iron and protein for the healthy growth of the foetus. Calorie needs may increase by 20-25 percent, reaching 2,500-2,700 kilo calories. These increased needs are vital to the growth of the bones, teeth, cells and metabolism of the foetus, and insufficient supplements may result in osteomalacia in the mother, or rickets or chondropathy in the baby after birth. Similarly, such ailments can be checked by administering calcium prescriptions combined with vitamin D. However, it will be much better for them to eat more eggs, kelp, soybeans, animal liver, edible fungus and fruits. This not only improves the appetite of the pregnant mother, but also prevents the occurrence of the above malnutritional ailments, including congenital deformity of the foetus.

Nutrition for the lactating mother is of vital importance too. Up to 2,000 ml of mother's milk may be secreted per day, containing the protein, inorganic calcium, phosphorus, iron, fats, iodine, etc., essential to the newborn infant's growth. It is clear that the mother's diet serves a dual purpose, providing for both mother and infant's nutritional needs. It is also preferable for lactating mothers to take their nutrients from food rather than from drugs.

Similarly, menopausal women need more nutrition as compared to males of the same age. They need a more nutritious diet rich in protein, iron, and vitamins to cope with the increasing demands from physiological and psychological changes due to hormonal disturbances.

3. For the elderly

Old age is characterized by a progressive degeneration of mental and physical capacities, such as lowered concentration, forgetfulness, non-persistence, low metabolic rate, low eating capacity, emaciation, decrease of hypodermic fat tissues, low digestive power, and low resistance to diseases. All these are irresistible natural changes. What we can do is to delay the onset and slow down the process of senility. To attain this goal, comprehensive measures are needed, of which dietotherapy is one important part.

For the elderly, it is advisable to administer easily digested, non-greasy and delicate, rather than rough, foods. They should be encouraged to take more foods with a high fibre of cellulose content, helpful to overcoming senile habitual constipation. It is also advisable not to take too much high calorie foods, such as butter, cheese or chocolate, since the elderly are usually less active and so consume less energy. Unrestricted food taking would result in too much energy intake, which would, in turn, transform into fatty tissue deposited in the body, resulting in overweight and putting an excess burden on the heart. It is understandable, therefore, that striving for a reasonable diet regimen for the elderly also implies the prevention of diseases and a prolongation of life.

As a rule, the elderly are mostly liable to be in a deficient state, especially deficient in vital energy, so their food should be mainly nourishing in nature, however, easily digestible, and thus readily absorbed and assimilated. Traditional Chinese medicine recommends that these foods should be plain, benefiting and warm in nature, nourishing and beneficial to the kidney to make up for the universal shortage of fluids and seminal fluid in the elderly.

4. For special professionals

In modern society, the division of labour yields professionals in a great variety of fields. Workers in different professions have different nutritional needs, due to the demands of their working conditions. Neglect of such special needs can eventually result in physical defects or even severe ailments over a long period of development.

Due to limitations of space, it is impossible to introduce all the special dietary requirements for each profession. Here, only special medicinal diets for athletes, white-collar workers and workers on night shift are briefly introduced.

From a medical point of view, athletes are characterized by a very high energy consumption. During activity, the muscles are violently contracted and a state of high mental concentration is maintained. Some activities demand an even greater burden of energy consumption, such as weight-lifting, which requires a huge consumption of oxygen and energy. When the muscles contract vigorously, the normal process of glycogen decomposition and oxygen supply lag behind physiological demand, creating a state of "debt". Hence, they need a special supply of high nutrition foodstuffs, including milk and its side-products, eggs, lean meat, chicken, animal viscera, sea foods, fruits, chocolate, beans, etc. Since their digestive functions are highly active and metabolism high, greasy foods are feasible for these special professionals.

For white-collar workers, though they do not perform much muscular activity, the energy and oxygen consumption of brain cells is several times higher than that of other cells in the body. Hence, they too need foods of a high nutritional and energy value. Foods which have the action of activating blood circulation and eliminating stagnancy are also highly recommended, such as root of herbaceous peony (*paeonia loetiflora*), hawthorn, woo-long tea, etc. These foods and drinks have been shown to be quite helpful in preventing blood stagnation, which is common in white-collar workers due to their lack of physical exercises, making them susceptible to thrombosis or arteriosclerosis formation.

For those workers on night shift, aside from taking nutrition similar to common workers, emphasis should be put on the supply of food rich in vitamin A, such as carrot (rich in carotene, the precursor of vitamin A), animal liver, sweet potatoes, etc. This is simply because night shift workers work under artificial light and consume much more vitamin A. If such consumption is not supplemented in time and in sufficient amounts, certain kinds of diseases, such as night blindness, are liable to occur.

V. MEDICINAL FOODS FOR COMMON DISEASES

As mentioned above, one of the unique contents of traditional Chinese medicine is the basing of its treatment on the differential diagnosis of symptoms and signs. The nature of the disease, either deficient or excessive, cold or heat, superficial or interior, should first be determined and treatment is then given on the basis of such diagnosis. The process for dietotherapy is the same. Below are some of the medicinal foods recommended for certain common diseases.

1. Common cold

In traditional Chinese medicine, the common cold is divided into two types, cold-wind and hot-wind, which should be treated with different medicinal foods.

Cold-wind type: Manifestations are fever, chill without perspiration, headache, pains over the whole body, obstruction of nose (stuffy nose), nasal secretion (runny nose), white coating tongue, mildly quick pulse. Prescriptions:

a. Decoction of ginger with sugar: 25 g of ginger, cleaned and sliced into small chips, then put into a bowl. Add boiling water and cover for 5-10 minutes. Add an equal amount (25 g) of brown sugar. Drink the decoction while hot, then cover oneself up well, sleep and get sweating.

b. Decoction of scallion and ginger: Scallion stalk and fresh ginger, 25 g each. Cut into small pieces. Prepare a small bowl of bean starch vermicelli, or rice or flour noodles with salt. Add the scallion and ginger pieces and eat. Then cover oneself up well, sleep and get sweating.

Hot-wind type: Manifestations are high fever, no chill, slight sweating, thirst red eyes, sore throat, headache, slightly yellow coating tongue and rapid pulse. Prescriptions:

a. Chrysanthemum, peppermint and mulberry leaf drink: Chrysanthemum and mulberry leaves, 5 g each, bitter bamboo leaves and cogongrass root 30 g each, and peppermint, 3 g. Put all the ingredients in a bowl or cup, pour in boiling water and cover for 10 minutes. Drink the decoction like tea.

b. Peppermint sweets: Boil 500 g of cane sugar with a considerable amount of water at a low heat until it becomes sticky. Then slowly add 5 ml of peppermint powder or peppermint oil and stir steadily until the mixture sticks to the stirring implement like threads. Pour the sugar into a big porcelain tray (coated with a thin layer of vegetable oil). Cut the hardened sugar into small pieces. Take several times daily for a mild common cold.

2. Influenza (flu)

Generally known as "severe common cold". Its manifestations are sudden onset, severe headache and pain over whole body, congestion of the eyes and throat, coughing and high fever. It is highly infectious, usually affecting many people in the same area.

Prescriptions:

a. Thoroughly rinse and clean 250 g of turnip. Chop up, then immerse in vinegar for several hours. Eat with hot rice porridge.

b. Take soybeans 10 g, fresh coriander 30 g. Cook the soybeans in water for about 15-20 minutes, then add the coriander and boil for another 10 minutes. Eat the whole dose once daily.

c. Take tender peppermint leaves 3 g and licorice root 3 g. Put them together in a cup, pour in boiling water and cover for 15 minutes. Drink it hot, two or three times a day.

d. Take bean curd 200 g, processed (fermented) soybeans 12 g and scallion stalk, 15 g. Cook bean curd in water until it is well done. Add fermented bean and scallion stalk and boil for another 20 minutes. Eat it all while hot, then cover oneself up well, sleep and get slight sweating.

3. Bronchitis

This refers to chronic bronchitis, not acute bronchitis developing from a common cold, which is the result of long irritation of the bronchus. Its manifestations are coughing with sputum and with no or very mild fever or headache.

a. Take a reasonable amount of rock candy and a pear of about 200 g chopped into pieces. Put these two in a bowl or cup, and steam in a water bath for half an hour. Eat the whole dose once or twice a day for 1-2 weeks.

b. Pig's lung porridge: Take a whole pig's lung of about 500 g, rinse and bring to the boil. After skimming, boil for another half an hour, then remove the pig's lung and chop. Mix some of the soup and 100 g of chopped lung with 100 g of rice and 50 g seed of Job's tears, cooking gently until soup becomes glutinous, rice and lung well done. Add some salt, ginger, onion or other spices and serve. This porridge is good for chronic cough, emaciation, profuse sputum or sputum with blood.

c. Lily porridge: Take dried lily 30 g (or 60 g fresh lily), a reasonable amount of rock candy and rice 100 g. Boil the lily first for 15 minutes, then add the rice and cook at a low heat until it becomes glutinous. Add the rock candy and boil for a further short while.

This porridge is good for moistening the lungs and is indicated for chronic bronchitis. It is not suitable for acute common cold, or acute bronchitis.

d. Nuts preserved with honey: Boil 250 g of stir-fried sweet apricot-nuts in water for about an hour. Add 250 g of walnuts. Boil until almost dry, then pour in 500 g of honey, stirring continuously. Remove it from heat as soon as it boils.

This preserved medicinal sweet is good for general body weakness, and bronchitis with prolonged coughing and shortness of breath.

4. Infectious hepatitis

Apart from those with biliary stones or hemolytic jaundice, those icteric patients with low fever can be treated by this method.

a. Vinegar and bone soup: Take 100 ml of vinegar (best prepared from glutinous rice), fresh pig's bone (best vertebrae), 500 g, and brown and white sugar, 125 g each.

Smash up the bones with a hammer and immerse in the vinegar. Add both sugars and then boil for half an hour. After it has cooled, filter with gauze. Discard the residue and keep the strained liquid in a bottle. Administer according to different ages:

5-10 years	10-15 ml
11-15 years	20-30 ml
adults	30-40 ml

Three times daily after meals, one month for a course. Interrupt a week before another course begins. For chronic hepatitis, 2-3 courses may be needed.

b. Loach powder: Keep several live loaches in fresh water for 1-2 days to rid them of impurities. Bake in an oven at 100°C until dry. If one has no oven, it may be boiled, then dried over a stove. Grind into powder. Dosage: 10 g, three times a day. For children the dose may be reduced. One course lasts 12-16 days. For chronic patients, several courses may be needed.

c. River snail soup: Put 10-20 live river snails in fresh water for 1-2 days so they evacuate any internal impurities. Crack the shells and take out the flesh. Mix with a cup of yellow rice wine, then dilute with water and cook. Drink the soup, though the flesh can also be eaten. Take once daily for a period according to the reaction.

d. Chinese date porridge: Rinse 10-20 Chinese dates. Cook 100 g of rice, adding the dates when the water comes to the boil and simmer until it becomes a glutinous porridge. It should be eaten daily over an extended period. If Chinese date is not available, 30 g of Chinese wolfberry seeds may serve as a substitute, prepared in the same way.

5. Mumps (parotitis)

A kind of viral infection in which the salivary glands mainly the parotic gland, are affected. Its manifestations are swellings and pain at the subaural region, especially during mastication. Sometimes, when not well treated, the sexual glands, especially the testes, may be adversely affected.

a. Soak 50 g of red beans in water for 1-2 hours. A portion is then pounded in a mortar and applied locally. The rest of the beans should be well-cooked and eaten. It should be taken at each meal for one week or until the illness is cured.

b. Rinse 50 g of fresh (or 20 g dry) day-lily and soak in water for 1/2 hour, then bring to the boil and simmer for 20 minutes. Take all the day-lily and soup, once daily.

6. Dysentery

Dietotherapy alone should only be used in chronic cases. For acute cases, drug therapy should mainly be administered at the same time.

a. Green tea with honey: 5 g of green tea infused in boiling water and left to stand for 10 minutes. Add some honey and then drink before it is cold. Repeat 3-4 times daily.

b. Garlic: 10-15 g of fresh garlic, eaten either whole or crushed. Since it may irritate the mouth's mucous membrane, some other food may be taken at the same time. Generally, one head of garlic daily is enough. If taken crushed, 30-60 g of purslane may be first boiled to make a soup and then added. A little white sugar may also be added. Administer 1-2 times daily for half a month. The second course should be after one week's interruption.

c. Dark plum (Fructus Mume) decoction: Make a concentrated decoction with 5-6 pieces of dark plum. Best taken before meals. It can be prepared in paste form by boiling 5 kg of dark plum at a low heat until well done. Discard the stones and filter. Cook the filtrate until it becomes sticky. Then prepare it as bean-sized pills. Take 3-5 pills, twice daily.

d. Pomegranate peel: It shows a definite effect on chronic diarrhoea and dysentery. Rinse 20 g of pomegranate peel and boil it for thirty minutes. Add some brown sugar and then discard the residue. Drink one cupful, 2-3 times daily.

e. Turnip: Take 500 g of peeled turnip, rinse and slice. Add cane sugar and vinegar in adequate amount according to one's taste. Eat it as you like at meals.

f. Decoction of dried persimmon and brown sugar: Dry 500 g of dried persimmon over a low heat until scorched, then grind into powder and store in a bottle. Dosage: 10 g with some brown sugar, swallowed with warm water, twice daily. May be administered over an extended period.

g. Braised finless eel: 500 g of live finless eel, cleaned and cut into slices. First fry it and then add a little soy sauce, vinegar, garlic and brown sugar. Add a little water, ground ginger and starch. After starch becomes sticky, it is ready for serving.

h. Purslane decoction: Take 200 g of fresh purslane (itself a tasty wild vegetable), 10-20 g hyacinth flower and boil together for 15 minutes. The decoction can then be administered. Purslane may also be prepared in powdered form after drying. Take 5 g for each dose with sugar, twice daily.

7. Malaria

Acute malaria can be satisfactorily controlled by drugs, while for chronic cases, the following dieto-remedies are recommended.

a. Carambola drink: Squeeze 1 kg of carambola. Cook the juice over a low heat until it becomes sticky. After this paste has cooled, add 500 g of white sugar and store in a bottle. Dosage: 1 teaspoonful, thrice daily.

b. Wild duck soup: Prepare a wild duck of about 1 kg, discarding the viscera and feathers. Cook with several slices of ginger, dates, a little oil, salt and yellow rice wine. Eat the meat and drink the soup. May be eaten over 2 or more days. Effective for chronic malaria.

8. Iron-deficient anaemia

This is the commonest type of all anaemic disorders. The foods mentioned here are effective only for iron-deficient anaemia, not for other types.

a. Date and sheep's bone porridge. Take 1-2 crushed sheep tibial bones, and 20-30 pitted dates. Boil the bones for 1-2 hours over a slow heat. Make porridge with 100-200 g of rice and the dates. Mix these two and boil for a short time longer. This will do 2 or 3 doses. Take daily for half to one month.

b. Bean porridge with brown sugar. Take 100 g of glutinous rice, 20 pieces of Chinese dates, black bean, 30 g and brown sugar in sufficient quantity. Boil the rice with the black beans until glutinous porridge is half prepared, then the pitted Chinese dates are added. The brown sugar is finally added once the porridge is ready. This can be eaten everyday over a long period.

c. Spinach and pig's liver soup. Take 100 g of pig's liver, sliced, and 100 g of spinach cut into segments. Coat the liver with starch and put into boiling water. Then, spinach, spices and salt are added. Eat at one sitting.

d. Bean and date soup. Take mung bean 50 g, Chinese date 50 g and some brown sugar. Boil the dates and beans until well-cooked. Add the sugar and boil for a few moments more, then administer. This can be taken daily for half to one month.

e. Dried longan pulp and mulberry fruit soup. Boil 15 g of dried longan pulp with 30 g of mulberry fruit until the longan pulp swells. Discard the residue, and then add some honey when it has cooled. Take once daily. This may be taken over a fairly long period.

f. Date and auricularia auricula-judae (an edible fungus) soup. Take 30 g of auricularia auricula-judae, rinse and immerse in water for half an hour. Then boil with Chinese dates (30 pieces) until soft. Brown sugar is then added. Take once daily over a fairly long period of time.

9. Anaphlactic purpura

This ailment is characterized by skin rashes or petechial lesions, coupled with abdominal aches or joint pains. Prescriptions:

a. Peanut skin soup. Boil 30 g of peanut skins with 20-30 g of Chinese dates at a low heat until the dates are well done. Throw away the residue and drink the soup. Take once daily for 5-7 days.

b. Chinese date. Take 10 dates thrice daily for 1-2 weeks. They can also be prepared as a date drink. Take 250 g of Chinese date. Add 1,500 ml water and boil until the dates are swollen. Discard the stones and boil for another 40 minutes. Filtrate, add 300 ml more water to the residue and boil again for another 40 minutes. Filter again and discard the residue. Mix the two filtrates and concentrate it over a low heat to about 750 ml. Drink 250 ml, thrice daily. Effective when administered over a long period.

c. Date and barley soup. Add 500 ml of water to 500 g barley and 15 g Chinese date. Boil at a low heat down to 150 ml and drink it all. Take once daily for 1-2 weeks.

d. Thick soup of Chinese date and pig's skin. Take 500 g of pig' skin with all the hairs pulled out and rinse thoroughly. Add an appropriate amount of water and boil at a low heat to make a sticky soup. Then, add 250 g of Chinese date and continue to cook until the dates are well done. Add an adequate amount of sugar, white or brown. Eat at meals as you like as a side dish for any length of time. Also good for haemophilia.

10. Hypertension

Referring to primary or idiopathic hypertension, rather than hypertension secondary to other disorders such as nephritis, pheochromocytoma, etc.

a. Jellyfish and water chestnut soup. Desalt 125 g of jellyfish by soaking it in water for a whole day. Slice it and 375 g of water chestnut (with peel) into small pieces. Put them into 1,000 ml of water and simmer over a low heat until 3/4 of the water has evaporated. Filter and discard the residue. Drink the filtrate, 125 ml per dose, twice a day. It can be administered over a long period, and is good for lowering and stabilizing blood pressure.

b. Celery. Celery has a blood pressure lowering action and can be administered in many ways. Cut celery into small pieces and squeeze out the juice. Add sugar, either white or brown, and sip it as one would tea. Celery can also be prepared as a decoction or cooked with balsam pear and eaten as a side-dish at meals.

c. Honey. Also has a certain blood pressure lowering action and is effective at the early stage of hypertension. Dilute honey with water and sip it as one would tea.

d. Mung bean and kelp porridge. Take kelp and mung beans each 100 g. Boil the mung beans first until they "bloom". Add rice and kelp and simmer at a low heat until sticky. Best eaten in the evenings, it can be taken over a long period.

e. Garlic and mung bean soup. Take 100 g mung bean and garlic, one clove for each year until 50 cloves are reached for those older than 50 years of age. Peel the garlic cloves and put them, with the mung beans, into a bowl. Add 500 ml of boiling water, cover, and leave to infuse for 10 minutes. Sugar may be added to taste; then drink as one would tea.

f. Take a fresh pig's gallbladder, fill it with several cleaned mung beans, then hang it out to dry. When completely dry, remove the beans. Take 6-7 beans with water twice a day. Can be administered for a fairly long period.

g. Sea cucumber with crystal sugar. Rinse 30 g of sea cucumber and discard its internal viscera. Add crystal sugar and water and simmer at a low heat. Best taken before the midday meal, the whole dose once per day. This can be taken for a long course.

h. Water chestnut and turnip juice. Cut water chestnut and turnip into pieces, 750 g of each. Wrap in gauze and press out the juice. Add some honey and then bottle. Drink 1 cup of the juice 2-3 times daily. Make fresh juice everyday.

i. Fish-head and elevated gastrodia soup. Take a silver carp's head. After rinsing, put it in an earthenware pot with 12 g of elevated gastrodia, some Chinese onion, vinegar, water and salt. Cook for more than half an hour. Eat the fish head and soup. This can be eaten regularly.

11. Diabetes mellitus

Dietotherapy is a treatment of decisive significance in diabetes mellitus, which can be effectively controlled provided rational dietotherapy is provided.

a. Sweet potato leaves. Also called white potato or red potato leaves. Take 60 g of fresh leaves (30 g dry leaves) and 100 g of fresh white gourd's skin (or 12 g dry skin). Cut both into small pieces and boil. Drink in the same way as tea, for any length of time.

b. Chinese yam soup. Take 100 g of fresh Chinese yam (or 20 g dried yam) and 20 g of Chinese trichosanthes and boil. Drink a bowl of this soup daily for any length of time. This soup may be also prepared by adding a pig's pancreas to 200 g of fresh Chinese yam, then boiling with a little salt. Administer once daily, dividing it into 4 doses, but take care that it does not go off.

c. Dark plum drink. Infuse 15 g of dark plum in boiling water, then drink as one would tea.

d. Cowpea soup. Boil 50 g of cowpea plus pods for 20 minutes. Drink the soup and eat the peas. Administer once daily.

e. Mare's milk. Drink 125 ml of boiled mare's milk twice daily for any length of time.

f. Superior Chinese yam. Steam and peel 500 g of Chinese yam. Mix in a bowl with 150 g of flour to make a paste. Make small cakes from the paste, garnishing with nuts and preserved fruits. Steam the cakes for 20 minutes. Finally, coat with honey solution (the solution is prepared by mixing one spoonful of honey with 100 g white sugar and some pork fat and starch, then cooking well). One batch of cakes may last 2-3 days.

g. Pig's stomach porridge. Boil a pig's stomach of about 500 g until it is more than half done, and then cut it into slivers. Take rice and the slivered pig's stomach, 100 g of each, and cook in the original soup. Add Chinese onion, ginger and garlic before serving.

h. Braised gluten. Fry 250 g of gluten for a while and then add ginger and Chinese onion. Add one bowl of water and some salt. When well cooked, add starch solution and continue to cook until it becomes sticky, then serve.

12. Simple goitre

a. Kelp powder. Bake kelp and seaweed, 500 g of each, until dry. Grind into powder and take 10 g daily. 250 g may also be made into soup. Take daily for half a month.

b. Laver. May be prepared in many ways, for instance, as a soup, or stir-fried with other ingredients. About 10 g is enough per dose.

13. Nephritic edema

a. Pig's stomach and lotus seed soup. Thoroughly rinse a pig's stomach and stuff it with 40-50 lotus seeds with their sprouts removed. Sew up the stomach and then boil until well done. Add a little salt and monosodium glutamate. Serve in 2-3 doses. It may also be served in sliver form with lotus seeds. Sesame oil, Chinese onion and garlic may also be added.

b. Cogongrass root and red bean porridge. Rinse and boil 200 g of fresh cogongrass root (50 g if dried) for ½ hour. Discard the residue, then add 50 g of red beans and continue to simmer until the beans "bloom". Add 200 g of rice and cook until porridge becomes sticky. Take the porridge in 2-3 doses.

c. Calabash soup. Take 50 g of calabash with its pulp and seeds discarded, rind of water melon and white gourd, 30 g each, Chinese date, 10 g. Add 500 ml of water and boil at a low heat until 150 ml is left. Discard the residue and drink the soup once daily. Also good for preventing heat stroke.

d. Take a snakehead fish of about 500 g and 50 g of red beans. Clean and gut the fish with scales remained, stuffing its stomach with the beans. Wrap the fish in several layers of thick paper. Stick a piece of lead wire through the mouth of the fish, wind it around the body, then immerse it in fresh water. When the paper is soaked through, embed the fish in a charcoal fire until it is well done. Take it without salt in two doses, for seven successive days as a course.

e. Poria porridge. Pulverize poria into powder and use 15-20 g with a reasonable amount of rice to make a porridge. This can be eaten daily over a long period.

f. Porridge made from membranaceus astragali. Boil 30-60 g of fresh astragali at a low heat in 200 ml of water until 100 ml remains. Add 100 g of rice and some brown sugar and simmer until the rice is well done. Finally add a little tangerine peel powder, bring back to the boil, then it is ready. This porridge can be eaten in the morning or evening, though it is not suitable for those who are deficient, have a fine and quick pulse, and a red tongue.

g. Pig's liver and mung bean porridge. Make a porridge out of 50 g of mung beans and 100 g rice. Add 100 g of cleaned and chopped pig's liver. Boil the porridge for a little while until the liver is done. There is no need to add salt. This porridge can be eaten regularly.

14. Rheumatism of joints and cartilage

a. Job's tear porridge. 50 g of Job's tear is boiled at a low heat until it forms a sticky porridge. White sugar is added before taking. Administer once daily for one month.

b. Slender acanthopanax root bark liquor. Soak 50 g of acanthopanax root bark in water and then boil at a low heat. Pour off the decoction at ½ and 1 hour intervals (adding more water after the first time). Take 500 g of glutinous rice. After rinsing, add water and boil with the above acanthopanax decoction to make sticky rice. When cold, add some distiller's yeast and ferment to make rice liquor. Serve it as beverage at meal time.

c. Inkfish liquor. Take 2 dried inkfish with bones and put into 250 ml of Chinese yellow wine, then boil at a low heat until well done. Drink the wine and eat the inkfish. The amount of wine drunk should vary according to individual tolerance. Drink once or twice daily for several days. For patients with impaired functions of the heart, kidney and liver, it should be administered with care or contraindicated.

15. Vertigo (Meniere's syndrome)

a. Gingko with Chinese date soup. 25 g of gingko's flesh is pulverized after having been baked dry, then kept in a bottle. Boil 50 g of Chinese dates until 100 ml of water remains. Take 5 g of gingko powder, swallowed down with 30 ml of the date soup, thrice daily for 1 week.

16. Epilepsy

a. White (or black) pepper corns and dried turnip are combined in a 1:2 ratio and ground into powder, then kept for administering. Swallow 2 g with warm water thrice daily. This may be administered for a long period. However, an anti-epileptic drug should be administered at the same time when the seizures occur, while this food is good at consolidating the treatment and can be administered for more than a year.

b. Olive-alum cake: Take 5,000 g of pitted olive and crush in a mortar. Boil at a low heat until sticky. Add some alum powder. By this time the weight should be about 1/5 of the original. Store in a bottle. Dilute with water and drink twice daily, 1 spoonful (15 g) each time. Sugar may be added. A month period of interruption is needed if a second course is to be begun.

17. Headache

a. Thick soup of elevated gastrodia tuber with pig's brain. 10 g of elevated gastrodia tuber is boiled with a whole pig's brain for 1 hour at a low heat. Discard the herbal residue and eat the brain and soup at one draught or divide into doses. This soup can be administered often and is good for migraine and nervous headaches.

b. Feather cockscomb seed drink. Soak 300 g of feather cockscomb seed in water and then boil at a low heat. Drain off the water after 20 minutes and then add more water. Repeat this process twice more. Mix the three solutions and concentrate by simmering until it becomes sticky. When cooled, add 400 g of white sugar, mix thoroughly and dry in the sun. Then pulverize it into powder and keep in a bottle. Administer in 10 g doses dissolved in hot water, thrice daily.

18. Diarrhoea: Referring to those chronic diarrhoea without distinct special causes

a. Pomegranate skin and honey paste. Cut 1,000 g fresh pomegranate skin (half weight if dried) into small pieces and boil in water at a low heat. Drain off the liquid at ½ and 1 hour intervals adding more water as required. Mix the 2 solutions and concentrate by simmering until sticky. Add 300 g of honey. Once it has returned to the boil, remove from the heat and let it cool. Take in hot water two or three times a day.

b. Lotus seed cake. Take 50 g of lotus seed with sprouts discarded. Boil at a low heat until soft, then pound into a paste. Cook some rice, either regular or glutinous, and mix it with the paste. When thoroughly mixed add white sugar, then administer.

c. Pig's kidney thick soup. Take a pair of cleaned pig's kidneys and cut into small pieces after cutting away the white tissue of each piece. Add 12 g of rhizoma drynariae and some water. Cook for 1 hour at low heat, then add some salt and flavouring. Take in one draught or 2 doses. This diet may be taken for 1-2 weeks, and is effective for chronic, prolonged and diarrhoea before dawn.

d. Lichee porridge. Crush 50 g of dry lichee flesh with 16 g each of lotus seed and Chinese yam in a small mortar. Add water and cook until well done. Rinse 200 g of rice, add the above crushed ingredients and sufficient water and cook until the rice is well done. Administer each evening. This is good for diarrhoea before dawn.

e. Gorgon fruit powder. Pulverize 50 g of peeled gorgon fruit. Rinse 100 g of rice, add the powder and sufficient water and cook until the rice becomes sticky. Good for chronic diarrhoea.

19. Allergic asthma

a. Egg and turnip. Around the winter solstice, take a turnip (red skin with white flesh) and cut into two equal pieces. Cut a small hole in each half in such a way that when the halves are put together, an egg may be placed in the hole with the rounded end facing upward. Then put a whole egg inside and bind the turnip together with string. Plant the turnip in a flowerpot. Give attention to water, sunlight and temperature to ensure its growth. Eighty-one days after the winter solstice, take the egg out carefully. It should not be rotten, although the yolk may be scattered through the egg white. Cut the turnip into slices, cook for a while and then add the egg and cook for a little longer. No salt should be added. Divide into two doses, taken in one day. Several doses should be prepared at a time, in case any of the eggs goes rotten and should not be used.

b. Gingko. Cook 12 g of gingko flesh in water for 20 minutes. Then add honey or white sugar and drink. Administer once daily. Interrupt after 1 week's dosage. Not suitable for children.

20. Intestinal obstruction due to ascariasis

This ailment mostly occurs in children. For frequent discharging of worms in faeces, severe abdominal pain, vomiting with ascaris or even faecal material, the following dietotherapy is recommended.

a. Sesame oil (peanut oil or rapeseed oil may be substituted). Add the juice squeezed out of 50 g of the white portion of Chinese onion to 500 ml of oil. For children under 15, administer 20 ml every 6 hours, three times in all. For adults double the dosage.

b. Peanut oil. Boil the oil. After it has cooled, drink a cupful (100 ml), 3 successive doses at 6 hour intervals. Half doses for children.

Note: After the abdominal pains have disappeared, an anthelmintic should be administered.

21. Alcohol poisoning

a. 15 g of tea infused in boiling water for 10 minutes. Drink a large cupful.

b. Put 15 g of white sugar in 30 ml of vinegar. Dilute with hot water, and when the sugar has completely dissolved, drink.

c. Take 60 g of black soya beans. Add a suitable amount of water and heat until boiling, then drink.

22. White hair

Refers to white hair in youngsters. However, it is also good for delaying the appearance of white hair in the elderly.

a. Multiflower knotweed tuber porridge. 30 g of this tuber is boiled in an earthenware pot until a concentrated solution is left. Meanwhile, 100 g of rice is cooked and several dates and some rock candy added. Pour in the tuber solution and continue to cook until it becomes sticky. Eat every morning and evening. Do not use iron pots. Contraindicated for chronic diarrhoea.

b. Chinese wolfberry seed porridge. Cook 100 g of rice and 30 g of this seed until sticky. Take twice a day, morning and evening, and can be taken over a long period.

c. Honey paste for blackening hair. Ingredients include processed multiflower knotweed tuber, 200 g; poria, 200 g; angelica sinensis, 10 g; Chinese wolfberry seed, 50 g; Chinese dodder seed, 50 g; bidentate achyranthes root 50 g; fructus psoraleae, 50 g; and black sesame, 50 g. Soak all the ingredients in water for ½-1 hour, and then boil. Pour out the solution three times, once every 20 minutes, adding more water each time. Mix these three portions and boil at a low heat until it becomes gelatinous. Add an equal amount of honey. Stir thoroughly and boil. Then let it cool down for·use. Take 1 teaspoonful twice daily, morning and evening.

d. Black sesame porridge. Grind 25 g of black sesame. Cook with 150-200 g of rice to make porridge. This can be taken for a long period.

23. Insomnia

Insomnia patients should not take sleeping pills for a long time so as to prevent drug tolerance or dependence. The advantage of dietotherapy for insomnia is that it can be used persistently without side-effects.

a. Wild jujube seed porridge. 30-45 g of wild jujube seed, either raw or cooked, is crushed and boiled to make a thick soup. Cook 100 g of rice, adding the soup when the rice is half done, then boil until well done. This porridge can be administered for a long course.

b. Mulberry fruit honey paste. Rinse 1 kg of fresh mulberry (a half dose if dried) and boil in water. Pour out the solution after 30 minutes. Add more water and boil for another 30 minutes. Pour out the solution, to which the first solution is then added. Simmer this mixture until it becomes sticky, then add 300 g of honey and bring back to the boil. Let it cool and store in a bottle for use. Take a teaspoonful, twice daily. The fruit may also be directly boiled with honey at a low heat to make a preserved fruit for administering.

Pig's kidney with angelica root, codonopsis pilosula root, and Chinese yam. Clean 500 g of pig's kidney by cutting away the white tissues. Put it in a container and add 10 g each of angelica root, codonopsis pilosula root and yam. Add some water and cook until kidney is well done. Take out the kidney and cut into small pieces, cutting rhomic check on the surface. Add flavouring, ginger, garlic and sesame oil and take it in a draught.

24. Dyspepsia

Referring to abdominal distention belching, and regurgitation after meals.

a. Pig's stomach porridge. Thoroughly rinse a pig's stomach of about 500 g and boil in water until 70-80 percent done. Slice it into threads. Then add to 200 g of rice and cook until porridge is well done and sticky with the pig's stomach completely done. Take it in 2 doses. This porridge may be administered for a long period.

b. Preserved hawthorn. 500 g of pitted hawthorn is put in a pot and cooked in water until nearly dry. Then add 250 g of honey and cook again at a low heat until well done. Store in a pot. Effective for dyspepsia due to over-eating of meat, weakened spleen and stomach or diarrhoea. Also good for coronary heart disease.

c. Shredded turnip cake. Cut a turnip into slivers. Stir-fry it with vegetable oil and add minced lean pork with a few drops of sesame oil and some mono-sodium glutamate. Make thin sheets of dough with flour, then wrap up the turnip mixture in them and bake. Eat the cakes as one likes.

d. Spleen benefiting cakes. Wrap up 6 g of dry ginger and 30 g of large-headed atractylodes root in gauze and boil with 250 g of Chinese date for about 1 hour. Discard the gauze and continue to cook until the dates are well done. Discard the stones. Take 15 g of the ground inner layer of hen's gizzard, to which 500 g of flour is added. Bake cakes with the flour sheets. It is good for children's dyspepsia.

e. Sugar preserved kumquat. Take 500 g of kumquat and press into flat cakes in a clean container. Discard the pips. Immerse the cakes in 250 g white sugar (dissolved in a little hot water for 24 hours). Then heat slowly until the sugar becomes dry. Add another 250 g of white sugar, cover with gauze and wait several days before using.

f. Spiced rice crust. Take 60 g of rice crust*. Add cinnamon cassia bark, fructus amomi, pericarpium zanthoxyli, fennel fruit and thizoma atractylodis, each 6 g, and grind into powder. Store the powder in a bottle. Dosage: 3-6 g, twice a day (only yellow crust can be used; scorched crust is not applicable).

g. Take 500 g of rice crust and fry until yellow. Mix with scorched hawthorn 60 g, Chinese yam 120 g and fructus amomi 30 g, then grind into powder and store in a bottle. Take 10 g per dose, twice daily. White sugar may be added.

---

*Rice crust is the yellow crust left on the bottom of a pan when rice is slightly overcooked.

25. Impotence

a. Herba cistanchis porridge. Put 15-30 g of herba cistanchis into an earthenware pot with water and boil until quite well done. Discard the residue. Make porridge with 100-150 g of rice; 100 g of mutton may also be added. Add some ginger, bring back to the boil, then it is ready for use. Contraindicated in chronic diarrhoea.

b. Fried chives and walnut. Deep fry 50 g of walnut in vegetable oil. Then fry some chives until about 80 percent done. Mix the two ingredients. Add some salt and then serve at a meal.

c. Duck with Chinese caterpillar fungus. A male duck of about 1 kg is cleaned and viscera discarded, then boiled or steamed in an earthenware pot (or aluminium pot), with 10 pieces of Chinese caterpillar fungus, and some ginger, Chinese onion and flavouring added. First boil strongly and then simmer until well done. Add some salt and serve. Repeat every 2-3 days.

d. Sheep's kidney and Chinese wolfberry leaf porridge. Rinse 500 g of Chinese wolfberry leaves and cut into small pieces. Clean a pair of sheep's kidneys as usual and then cut into pieces. Take 200 g of rice to which the above ingredients are added and then cook at a low heat until well done. Add some salt, Chinese onion and ginger pieces. This diet can be taken often.

e. Fry 200 g of balsam pear seeds and then grind into powder. Store in bottle for use.

Dosage: 10 g twice daily for ten days. Swallow with yellow rice wine.

26. Hiccup

a. 15-30 g of sword beans with pods are boiled in 200 ml of water. Add 3 pieces of ginger. Boil until half the volume remains. Add some brown sugar. Drink the soup in 2-3 doses within one day.

b. Put 3 g of clove and 10 g of orange peel in water. Boil for ½ hour and drink the solution.

c. Rinse 30 g of fresh ginger and crush in a mortar, squeezing out the juice, to which 30 ml of honey is added. Take 1 teaspoonful, 2-3 times daily.

d. Bake 50-100 g of dry lichee, including stones and skin. Then grind into powder. Swallow 10 g with water, twice daily.

e. Fry 6 g of dried inner layer of hen's gizzard. Grind it with salt into powder. Dosage: 3 g, thrice daily. Swallow with water.

27. Epistaxis (nasal bleeding)

Referring to nasal bleeding which occurs without obvious causes and cannot be cured by ordinary methods.

a. White turnip juice. Rinse 500 g of white turnip and cut into small pieces. Wrap with gauze and press to obtain juice. Take 50 ml and add white sugar before drinking. Administer thrice daily.

b. Steamed lotus root and rice cake. Take lotus root powder, rice powder and white sugar, each 250 g. Mix them with an appropriate amount of water to form a paste and steam. Take as many as one likes, two or three times daily.

28. Habitual constipation

Referring exclusively to constipation without obvious causes, not including that due to high fever or obstruction by tumour mass, etc.

a. 500 g of sweet potato is rinsed and cut into medium pieces, then cooked. Add salt or white sugar before eating. Administer before going to bed every evening for 15 successive days.

b. Cut 100 g of white turnip into pieces. Press to obtain juice. Add 50 ml of honey. Administer once daily.

c. Stir-fry equal amount of walnut and sesame and grind into powder. Take 1 teaspoonful (about 20 g) every evening before bed time. This may be taken with some honey.

d. Cut 1 kg of fresh potato into small pieces and press out the juice. Boil this juice until it becomes sticky. Add an equal amount of honey and boil again until it is concentrated like honey itself. Remove from heat and store in bottle when cool. Dosage: 1 teaspoonful, twice daily before meals or before bed time.

e. Take 250 g of Chinese trichosanthes fruit and discard the flesh, then put in an earthenware pot with a suitable amount of water and 100 g of white sugar. After boiling at a low heat, stir into paste to be used as filling. Then make a dough out of flour (750 g), yeast and water. Once risen, roll out into cakes and stuff with the filling, then either steam or bake and serve as a staple food.

f. Cut up an onion of about 100 g into slices. Another 100 g each of white turnip and potato are also cut into slices. Stir fry the above slices and serve at a meal.

29. Hoarseness

Referring only to hoarseness due to common cold rather than severe laryngitis.

a. Clean and peel a pear and press out the juice. From time to time drink a mouthful of juice, keep it in the mouth, then swallow it drop by drop.

b. Cut up 30 g of old, salted and dried leaf mustard. Boil for a short while. Drink the soup, keeping it in the mouth and swallow bit by bit. Take twice or thrice a day.

c. Soak 50 g of raw peanuts in cool water for a whole night. Discard the membranes and cook over a low heat in an aluminium pot until soft. Administer once daily.

d. Olive. Rinse some olives and keep one in the mouth, swallowing the saliva. Repeat according to the condition.

e. Take slices of fresh white turnip. Dosage: 5-10 slices, thrice daily.

f. Press the juice from a fresh turnip and some fresh ginger. Mix the juices, keep in the mouth, then swallow drop by drop.

30. Enuresis (bed-wetting)

a. A complete set of hen's intestines is thoroughly cleaned and then baked dry. Grind into powder and add some white sugar. Take after dinner with hot water for three successive days.

b. Cake of cock's intestine. Make cock's intestine powder as above. Then mix with 250 g of flour and add some water to make a soft dough. Add some vegetable oil and salt, then bake as cakes. Administer every evening, one set of intestines sufficient for two doses.

c. Poria and yam steamed stuffed bun. First steam poria and Chinese yam, each 100 g and then make a paste. Mix this with 200 g of flour and 300 g of white sugar to serve as the skin of the bun. Use white sugar, preserved fruits and preserved plum slivers as the stuffing. Make steamed buns and administer for a 1-2 week period.

31. Night sweating

a. Membranaceous milk vetch root porridge. Make a concentrated solution of this vetch by boiling 30-60 g of the raw material in water. Add some brown sugar and 100 g of rice and make a porridge. When done, add a little tangerine peel. This porridge can be administered for a long period.

b. Put 250 g of pork (preferably abdominal wall portion) in 500 ml of rice wine and cook at a low heat until well done. Add some white sugar. Administer once every two or three days.

c. Eight pig's trotters (half dose for children) are rinsed thoroughly and boiled. Once boiling, simmer at a low heat until the soup becomes thick. Take in a draught. Administer once daily for 3 successive days.

d. Measure 125 g of fresh, cleaned loach, then first fry in oil until yellowy-red and simmer in 500 ml of water until 150 ml is left. Add ginger slivers and salt. Take in a draught (eating both fish and soup), once daily for 3 days. For children, it may be taken in 2-3 doses.

e. Soak 150 g of black soybeans in 500 ml of water for a few hours. Take 9 g of dried bean skin. Mix 9 g of floating wheat (put the wheat in water, use those grains which float on the surface of the water) with the bean skin and cook to make a soup. Take it in a draught. 9 g of membranaceous milk vetch root may also be used, in which case the floating wheat should be reduced to 3 g.

f. Make a soup out of the spongy core of maize, and drink. Good for sweating due to deficiency in postpartum women.

g. Take 120-150 g of the crust which remains on the sides of the pot when cooking beancurd. Boil this crust and drink the soup and the residue.

h. Take Chinese date and black plum, each 10 pieces and make a decoction. Administer morning and evening, twice daily for 10 days.

i. Make a decoction from 12 g of mulberry leaves which have suffered frost. Take the decoction once daily for 10 days.

32. Urticaria (nettle rash)

a. Divide a bundle of Chinese chives into two halves. One half is cooked for eating and the other crushed in a mortar. Then add some salt and apply locally.

b. Cut 50 g of dried taro stem into small pieces and boil in water at a low heat for ½ hour. Add some crystal sugar and boil for a while. Eat the whole solution with residue once daily for several days.

c. Boil 15 g of maize hair for 20 minutes. Discard the residue and add 100 g of sweet fermented glutinous rice and bring back to the boil. Add some white sugar and drink.

33. Mastitis

a. Squeeze out the juice of an orange. Add a teaspoonful of yellow rice wine. Mix the two ingredients. Dilute with cool boiled water. Take twice daily, in the morning and evening, using one orange each time.

b. Grind 30 g of Chinese trichosanthes to which 100 ml of yellow rice wine is added. Steam in a water bath at low heat for 20 minutes. Take warm, 20 ml per dose, twice a day.

c. Take 30-50 g of acanthaceous indigo tuber. Simmer in 250 ml of water until only 100 ml is left. Add some yellow rice wine and drink in a draught. Also crush a fresh tuber with salt and add some vinegar to make a paste for local application, once daily.

d. A cup of sweet fermented glutinous rice is warmed. Mash some chrysanthemum leaves and press out the juice. Mix the two and drink. Also, mix some fermented glutinous rice with the chrysanthemum pulp and apply locally, twice daily.

e. Grind 50 g of deer antler into fine powder. Take 3 g with yellow rice wine, twice daily.

34. Leukorrhagia

Referring to profuse vaginal discharge. The following therapies are not indicated for leukorrhagia due to trichomonads.

a. Pork and inkfish soup. Rinse and treat 2 fresh inkfish of about 300 g and discard their bones and viscera. Cook with 250 g of lean pork. Add some salt and flavouring. Take once daily for 5 days.

b. Rinse 250 g of fresh lotus root and put in an earthenware pot with about 1 litre of water. Cook until only 7-800 ml is left and drink the soup. Repeat for 7 days as a course. It is good for sticky, yellow leukorrhagia.

c. Baked egg. Take 10 hen's eggs, make a small hole in each, and pour in 10 g of white pepper powder. Then enclose the whole egg with dough and bake the eggs on coals until well done. Take one egg daily for ten days as a course. An interval of 3-5 days should be allowed if a second course is necessary.

d. Cut 50 g of fresh Chinese chives into segments of 0.3 cm length. Immerse 30 g of dried scallop flesh in yellow rice wine for a while. Cook the scallop with the chives and take once daily.

e. Cook 30-60 g of crust from a pot used for cooking beancurd, an egg and 1 sheet of the skin of soybean milk together. Take before breakfast in one draught.

f. Bake dry 10 g of gingko flesh in an earthenware pot and then boil with some white sugar. Take the gingko flesh and the soup. One can also grind the flesh into powder and administer. Also, gingko powder may be put into an egg through a small hole in the shell. The hole is then covered with paper and the egg steamed. Take 1-2 eggs each day.

g. Boil 15 g of eggplant flowers with 30 g of *Smilax glabra* and drink once daily for a week.

h. Take sunflower stem and cut it and its core into pieces. Place 15-30 g in water and heat until it is just boiling. Take twice daily in the morning and evening.

i. Heat 20-30 g of dry broad bean flower in water until it boils for a while, then drink. Take daily.

j. Take the scales from two crucian carp or carp. Boil the scales at a low heat until it becomes sticky. Take with warmed yellow rice wine once daily for a week.

35. Dysmenorrhea

a. Hawthorn wine. Put 500 g of dried pitted hawthorn into a wine bottle. Add about 500 ml of Chinese white liquor (contains 60 percent alcohol). Cover tightly. Drink after 1-2 weeks. Take 10 ml, twice daily.

b. Put 100 g of cleaned saffron in a bottle. Add 400 ml of Chinese white liquor (60 percent alcohol). Leave to infuse for one week, shaking the bottle everyday. Take 10 ml each day.

c. Boil together 24 g of sliced fresh ginger, 9 g of Chinese prickly ash and 10 Chinese dates. Take in two doses every day for 1-2 weeks.

d. A sunflower disc (with seeds removed) of about 30-60 g is cut into small pieces and boiled for a short time. Add 30 g of brown sugar. Take in two doses every day, in the morning and evening.

36. Insufficiency of postpartum milk secretion

a. 2-4 pig's trotters are thoroughly cleaned and boiled at a low heat for more than 1 hour until done. Add a little salt and take (including soup) once daily. 9-12 g of pangolin scales or rice-paper plant may also be added to the soup during preparation.

b. Stew a fresh live crucian carp of about 120 g together with a pig's trotter until well done. Add some salt. Eat one or two pieces daily for 1-2 weeks.

c. Clean and scale a carp as usual. Add some water and onion segments, ginger shreds and salt. Steam or stew until done and eat (including soup).

d. Fry 250 g of black sesame over a low heat. Clean a pig's trotter as usual and stew to make a soup. Take 16 g of the sesame with the soup twice a day. The trotter should also be eaten.

37. Stopping lactation

Lactating women with profuse secretions of milk need dietotherapy when requiring the interruption of breastfeeding.

a. 200 g of barley, after rinsing, is covered with gauze and kept in a warm place. After sprouting, take 50 g of barley sprouts and boil. Drink 1-2 times daily for 1 week. The sprouts should be about 1-2 cm long.

b. Make wheat sprouts with 200 g of wheat in the same way as above. Fry the wheat sprouts until nearly scorched, then boil to make a soup. Drink daily in 3 doses for several days.

c. Stir-fry 60 g of wheat bran until yellow. Add 30 g of brown sugar. Mix thoroughly and fry again for a short while. Take several times a day. This recipe provides enough for 2 days.

d. Make a decoction from barley and wheat sprouts, each 60 g. Take in one day, divided into two doses for three successive days.

38. Fishbone stuck in the throat

a. Boil 10-20 black plums in an earthenware pot at a low heat until a concentrated solution is obtained. Drink a mouthful of solution and swallow it slowly drop by drop. The plum flesh may also be swallowed.

b. Take the gall-bladder of a mandarin fish and dry it in the shade. Grind into powder once dry and store in a bottle ready for use. Take 0.1-0.2 g and swallow with yellow rice wine.

c. Take an olive stone. Grind with water in a coarse porcelain pot. Swallow the juice.

39. Tuberculous lymph-adenitis

Referring to those mild cases without ulceration.

a. Pound up 500 g of taro. Also soak 500 g of jellyfish in water for a few hours. Then cut it and 500 g of water chestnut into small pieces and boil them together. Once well done, discard the residue, mix the soup with the taro paste and stir thoroughly. Bake until dry and keep in a bottle. Dosage: 3-6 g, 2-3 times daily, swallow with water.

b. Steam fresh taro until extremely well-done. Add some salt and soy sauce. Eat once every day as one likes. This may be taken for a considerable period.

c. Put 15 g of kelp, 15 g of seaweed and 50 g of dried lichee flesh in a pot with water and some yellow rice wine. Boil at a low heat until quite well done. Take the soup with all its ingredients once daily. It can be applied for a long time.

d. Put 50 g of oyster flesh in water and bring to the boil. Then add some garlic and salt. Serve at meals or with noodles. May be administered for a long period.

e. Put 7 lichee stones, 15 g of kelp and 15 g of seaweed in a pot with some water and yellow rice wine and simmer for more than 1 hour. Drink the soup once daily.

40. Chickenpox

a. Cut 100 g of carrot and 60 g of fresh coriander into small pieces and boil for a while. Discard the residue and drink the soup once daily.

b. Put 60 g of glycine soja and 60 g of red beans in a pot with some water and bring to the boil. Drink as a tea substitute, once daily.

41. Hyperlipemia (hypercholesteremia)

The following foods can be made into drinks to be taken regularly like tea:

a. Rhizoma of oriental water plantain, 6-9 g daily
b. tuber of multiflower knotweed
c. root of cogongrass
d. wild rice stem
e. *Alfal'fa*
f. the thick root of Chinese wolfberry
g. water chestnut
h. hawthorn.

Among them, items b, c, f can be administered in 12 g doses and made into drinks. The others can be eaten as vegetables.

42. Overweight

a. Leaves of oriental water plantain: 9-12 g of such leaves are put in a cup, infused with boiling water and left to stand for 15 minutes. Drink as a substitute for tea or coffee for a long course.

b. Cut up 250 g of celery and put in boiling water for 5 minutes. Once cooled, add some salt, monosodium glutamate and sesame oil. Chilli pepper may also be added. This food can be eaten as a side-dish every day for 2-3 months.

c. Take the spongy core of 3-5 maize rods and infuse in boiling water for several minutes. Take as a substitute for tea or coffee, twice daily. This may be administered for several months.

d. Every day eat non-refined grain, such as maize powder, Chinese sorghum, barley, sweet potato or brown rice, together with vegetables containing more cellulose (celery, horse radish, wild rice stem, bean curd, or other bean products). Eat mango or apple after meals every day. Perseverance (for at least 3 months) is of vital importance.

VI. COMMON MEDICINAL FOODS

As mentioned above, there is no sharp demarcation between medicines and foods. Some foods can be purchased from a drug store, some drugs from a grocery shop. Among these, some may be natural products and some artificial. Introduced here are more than 100 kinds of medicinal foods which are in common use and easily obtained. The items mentioned here are: its scientific Latin name (if available), nature and flavour, actions, indications, scientific chemical analysis and, last of all, therapeutic action.

A. Whole Plants

1. Onion

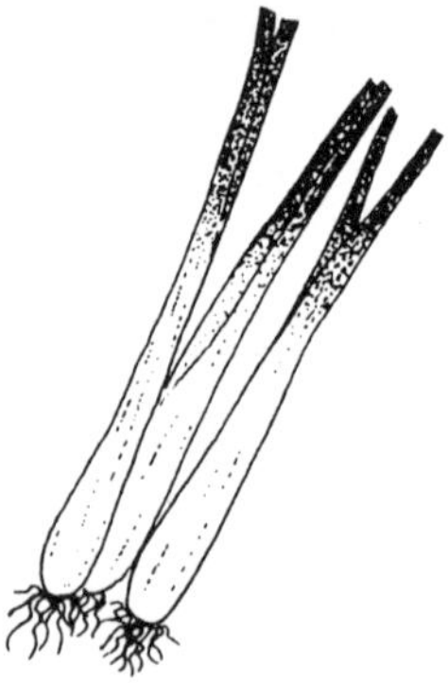

A herbaceous vegetable belonging to the lily family with many species, including the Chinese onion, onion, shallot, scallion, etc. In general the white portion, i.e., the bulb is used for medicinal purposes.

Nature and flavour: Pungent, warm, non-toxic.

Constituents: Carrotene, vitamins B_1, B_2, and C, calcium, iron, magnesium, volatile oil and allium.

Pharmacology: Diaphoretic, stimulating secretion of digestive juices, bactericidal action on dysentery bacilli.

Indications: Common cold, rhinitis. Also used locally for boils and carbuncles.

2. Garlic

A perennial plant of the lily family. The cloves of its underground bulb are used for medicinal purposes. A bulb with a single clove is preferred.

Nature and flavour: Pungent and warm with stimulating odour.

Constituents: Containing allicin, a volatile oil with stimulating odour. Also vitamins A, B, and C, cellulose, and minerals including calcium, phosphorus and iron.

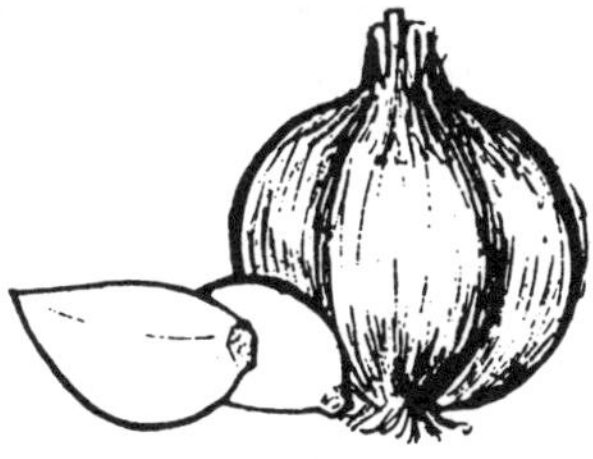

Pharmacology: Bactericidal action on typhoid fever, dysentery, cholera, diphtheria and pneumonia pathogens. Antitussive, and expectorant. Also a stomachic.

Indications: Dysentery (bacillary type) and prevention of epidemic meningoencephalomyelitis.

Note: Garlic should be used fresh (raw material). Cooked garlic is not effective. The maximum daily dose is one bulb. Since it is an irritant to the stomach, do not use in excessive doses. In traditional Chinese medicine, it is claimed that too much garlic is harmful to eye sight.

3. Coriander

A mono-rennial vegetable. The whole herb is used for medicinal purposes.

Nature and flavour: Pungent and warm with special fragrance.

Constituents: Volatile oil, fatty acid, decanal, nonahal, and linalool.

Pharmacology:

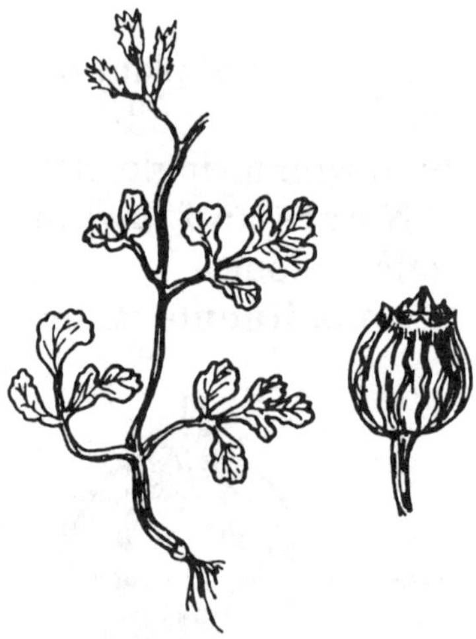

Helpful to the full eruptions of skin rash in measles and variola (German measles) which is recognized as a necessary sign for the smooth course of the disease. Promoting blood circulation and expelling evil-wind. Also an aromatic stomachic and detoxic.

Indications: Common cold, measles if the skin rash does not erupt smoothly. For measles, internal use and external washing may be applied simultaneously.

4. Chinese chives

A perennial vegetable of the lily family. The whole plant, seeds and root are used for medicinal purposes.

Nature and flavour: Pungent, sweet, warm and nontoxic.

Constituents: Containing volatile oil and sulphurous compounds, carrotene and vitamins B and C.

Pharmacology:

This is a stimulant, which promotes peristalsis of the intestines, with intra-intestinal antiseptic and bactericidal actions.

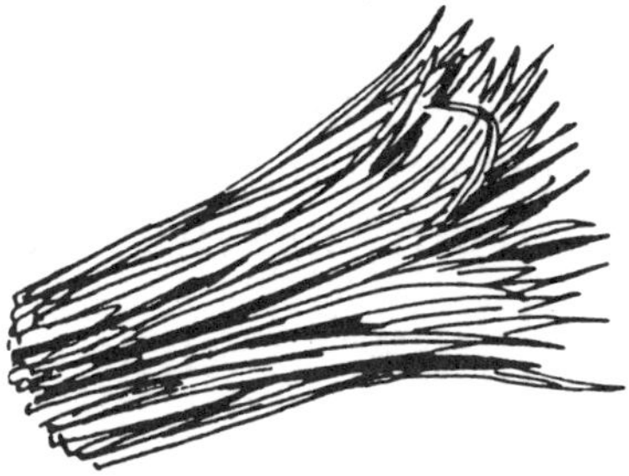

Action: The leaves activate the blood and eliminate the stagnant. The seeds have a strengthening and astringent action. The whole plant possesses the actions of activating blood and relieving stagnation.

Indications: Constipation, acute gastro-enteritis, dysmenorrhea and leukorrhagia.

Note: Contraindicated in patients of deficient vital essence with excessive evil-fire.

5. Celery

A vegetable belonging to the daucas family. There are two kinds of celery, watery and dry. The latter is commonly applied for medicinal purposes and is more aromatic.

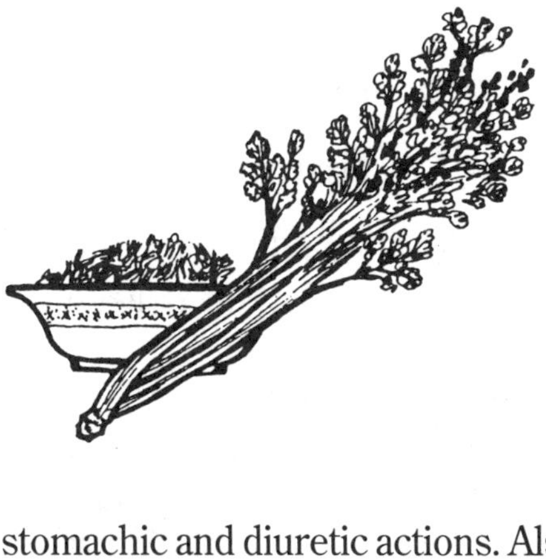

Nature and flavour: Sweet and cool.

Constituents: Containing glucoside of coriander, volatile oil, carrotene, vitamin C and a large amount of cellulose.

Pharmacology: Having sedative, stomachic and diuretic actions. Also the action of regulating menstruation.

Indications: Vertigo and headache due to hypertension, leukorrhagia and irregular menstrual cycles.

Note: Those with active peptic ulcer enteritis and dysentery should take with care.

6. Cogongrass Root

A plant belonging to the grass family with a white segmented root rich in water. The juice is sweet.

Nature and flavour: Sweet and cold.

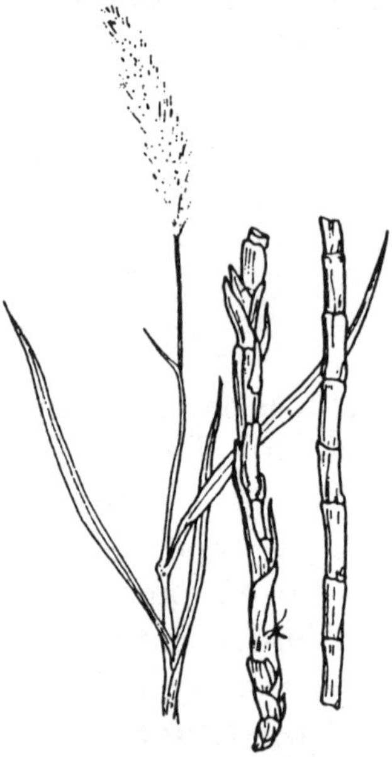

Constituents: Containing arandoin, cylindrin, glucose and steroids.

Pharmacology: Animal experiments show that cogongrass root possesses diuretic action, also with some antibiotic action.

Indications: The root is antipyretic with diuretic action and the flower cools the blood and has hemostatic action. It is applied for cases of hematuria, hemoptysis, acute nephritis and infections of the urinary system.

7. Spinach

A vegetable belonging to the chenopodiacea family. The whole plant is used for medicinal purposes.

Nature and flavour: Sweet and cold.

Constituents: Protein, cellulose, carrotene, vitamins B_1 and B_2 and C, oxalic acid, calcium, phosphorus, and high iron content.

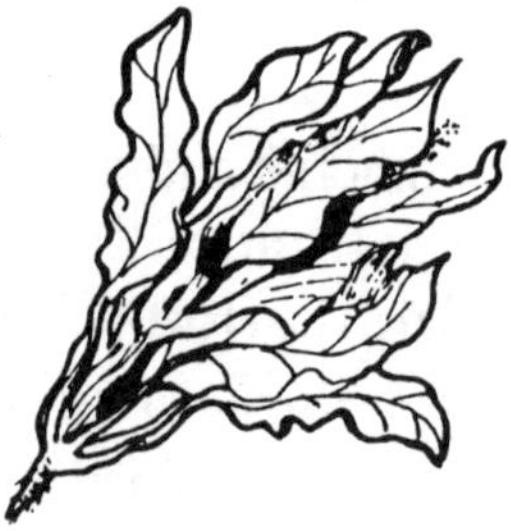

Indications: Iron-deficiency anaemia, hypertension and constipation. Also with some action on promoting digestion.

Note: Since it contains a considerable amount of oxalic acid, it is better to boil for a short while before administration to remove its puckery taste. Children should not eat too much spinach.

8. Purslane

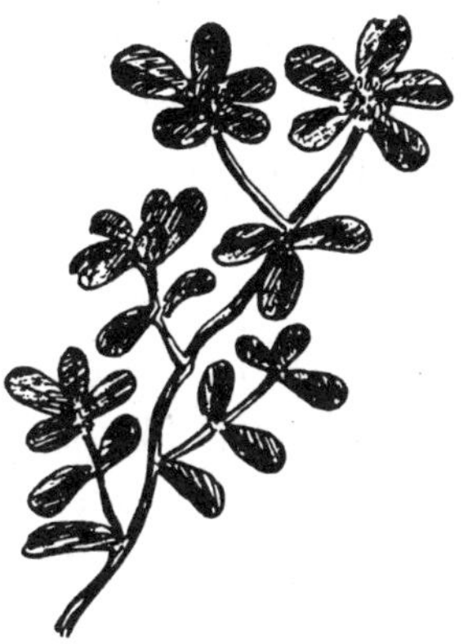

A plant belonging to the purslane family. The whole grass is used for medicinal purposes.

Nature and flavour: Sour and cold.

Pharmacology: Experiments prove it to have bacteriostatic action on bacillus E coli, typhoid and dysentery bacilli, especially on the latter.

Constituents: Noradrenaline, carrotene, vitamins B_1 and B_2, cellulose, calcium, phosphorus and iron.

Indications: Dysentery, enteritis. Also used as a subsidiary treatment for acute arthritis, and jaundice.

9. Peppermint

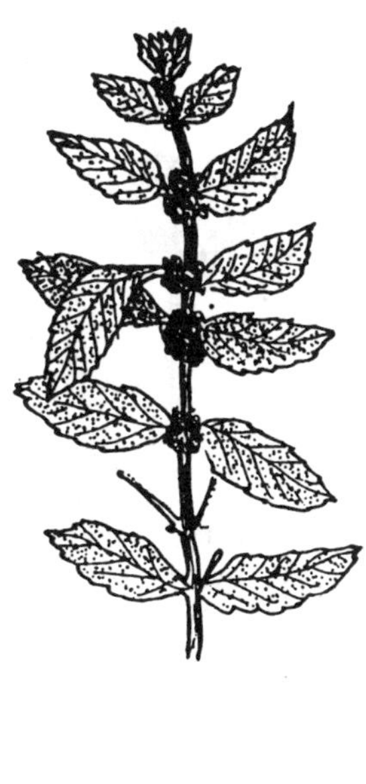

A plant belonging to the labiata family. The *longnau* peppermint produced in Suzhou, China is especially famous. The whole plant is used for medicinal purposes.

Nature and flavour: Pungent and cool.

Constituents: Volatile oil with menthol, menthone, limonene.

Pharmacology: The peppermint oil relieves spasms of the smooth muscles in the respiratory and alimentary tract. It also stimulates the peripheral nerve receptors for cold in the skin.

Action: Perspiration. Clearing the head and easing the eyes. Also having anti-heat stroke action.

Indications: Mainly applied in the first stage of the common cold. Also applied for skin pruritus or itching.

10. Capillary artemisia

A plant belonging to the composita family. Its young sprout can be served as a vegetable. It is collected in the 5th month (lunar calendar) and used as a medicine.

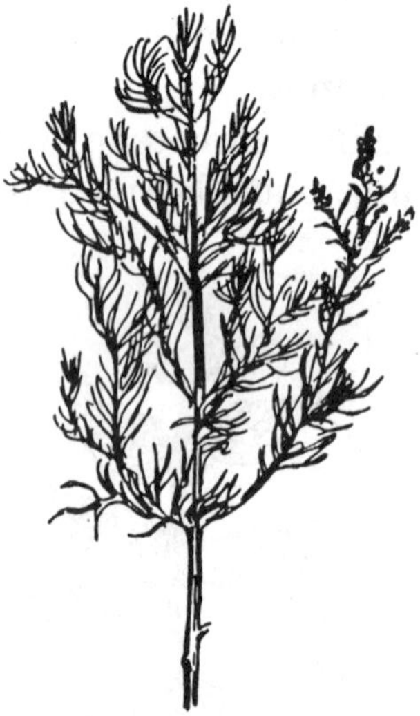

Nature and flavour: Bitter and slightly cold.

Constituents: Containing scoparon, caffeic acid, fatty acid and potassium chloride.

Pharmacology: In animal experiments, it reveals cholagogic action, lowering blood pressure, diuretic and antimicrobial actions.

Action: Antipyretic and expelling dampness in the body.

Indications: Commonly applied in infectious hepatitis (jaundice type), chole-cystitis and measles. Also used as a subsidiary treatment in hypertension, nephritis and liver cirrhosis.

11. Auricularia auricula-judae (an edible fungus)

Belonging to the auriculariae family with an ear-like appearance.

Nature and flavour: Sweet and moderate.

Constituents: Protein, fat and sugar. Also containing carrotene, vitamins B_1 and B_2, phosphorus, iron, calcium, steroid and phospholipids.

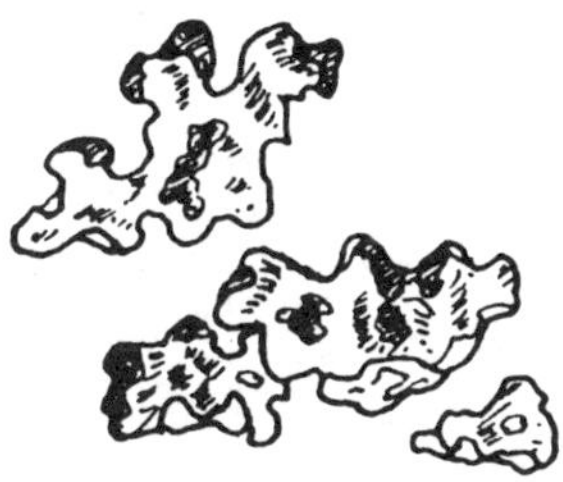

Action: Nourishing, benefiting blood. The white edible fungus has a stronger action than the black one. Also having some inhibitory action on tumour growth.

Indications: Anaemia, constipation. Also good for hypertension and vascular sclerosis.

12. Cinnamon bark

A plant belonging to the lauracea family. Commonly used as a flavouring for cooking.

Nature and flavour: Pungent and warm.

Constituents: Volatile oil, with cinnamaldehyde, cinnamone, cinnamic acid.

Action: Good for stomach ache of cold type. It possesses the action of warming the stomach. Also effective for abdominal distention and pains in the waist, knees and extremities due to cold.

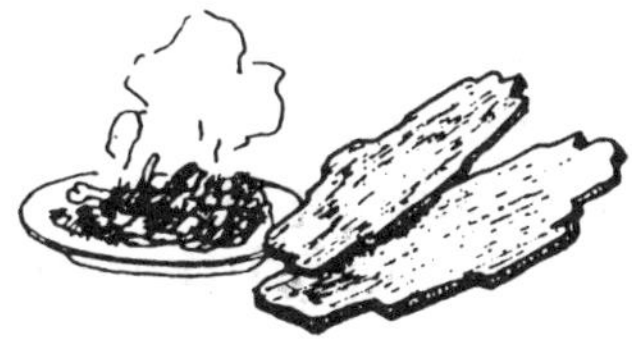

Indications: Stomach ache of cold type (manifestations include regurgitation of acid). Also good for postpartum women with lower abdominal and waist pains, leg pains and menstrual pains.

13. Tea

A perennial plant belonging to the camellia family. One of the most popular beverages in the world.

Nature and flavour: Sweet, bitter and slightly cold.

Constituents: Very complicated. Mainly containing caffeine, theophyline, cocaine, tannate, theobromine, geranial, vitamins B_1, B_2 and C, ergosteroid, volatile oil, theaspirone, etc.

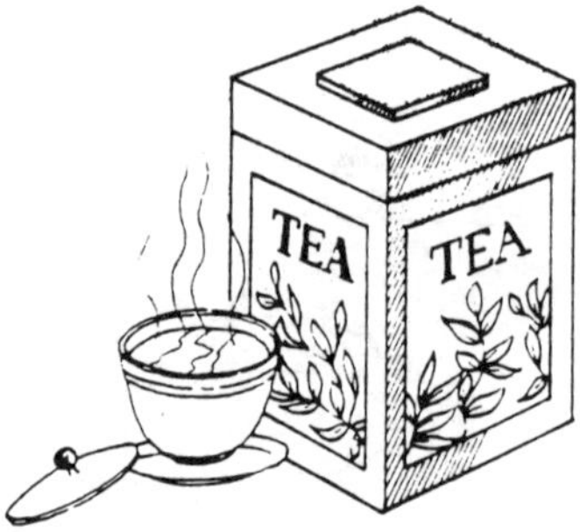

Pharmacology: Having the actions of stimulating the central nervous system, cardiotonic, diuretic, and astringency. Also an anti-toxic agent. The absorption of toxicity due to taking alkaloid and metallic salt can be delayed by taking concentrated tea solution. The tannin in tea promotes the health of capillaries, and decreases the tendency to bleeding.

Action: Antidote, stimulant, promoting blood circulation, anti-inflammatory and bactericide.

Indications: Bacillary dysentery, acute gastro-enteritis. It also can be applied locally in concentrated solution for herpes simplex or herpes zoster.

14. Seaweed

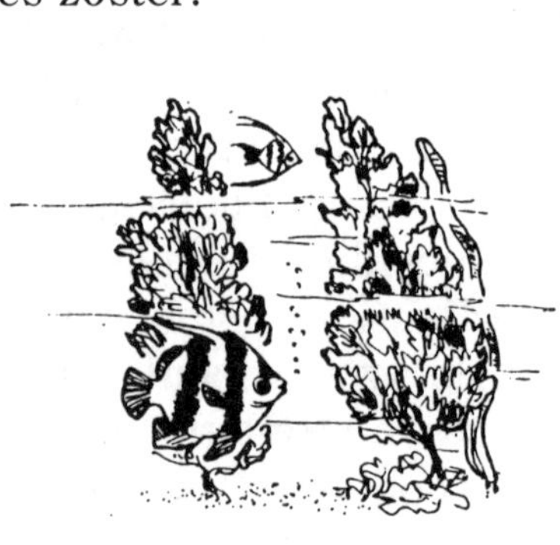

Belonging to the sagossum family.

Nature and flavour: Salty and cold.

Constituents: Sargassum fusiforame contains alginic acid, protein, mannitol, potassium and iodine. Sargassum pallidam contains alginic acid, protein, mannitol, potassium and iodine. Besides, it also contains sargassan, etc.

Pharmacology: In animal experiments, it reveals anti-coagulation action, lowering of blood fat and blood pressure actions. It also demonstrates temporary restraining of the rise of metabolic rate due to hyperthyroidism and is applied in the preparatory stage before thyroid operations. It also reveals inhibitory action on some tumours (erlich ascites cancer and uterine cancer).

Indications: Simple goitre, swelling of testes, lymphadenoma. For hypertension and arteriosclerosis it also reveals some inhibitory effect on the further development of the disease if administered at an early stage for a longer course.

15. Kelp

A kind of large edible alga now cultivated artificially on a large scale.

Nature and flavour: Salty and cold.

Constituents: Containing much iodine, also carrotene, vitamins B_1 and B_2 and protein.

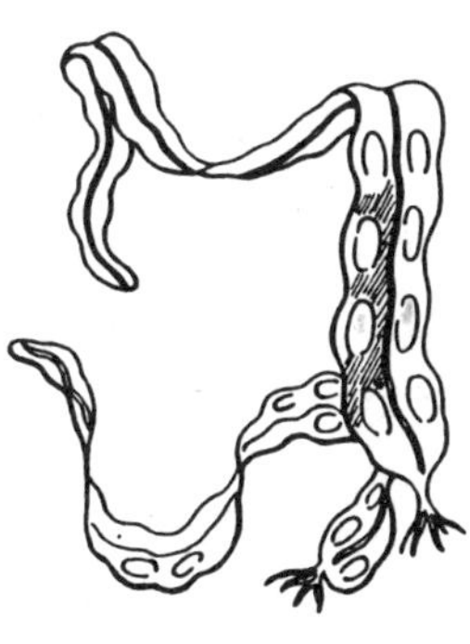

Pharmacology: The galacturonic acid in the protein has the action of lowering blood pressure. Its ether extract inhibits the growth of tuberculous bacilli.

Indications: Simple goitre, tuberculous lymphadenitis and chronic bronchitis in the elderly.

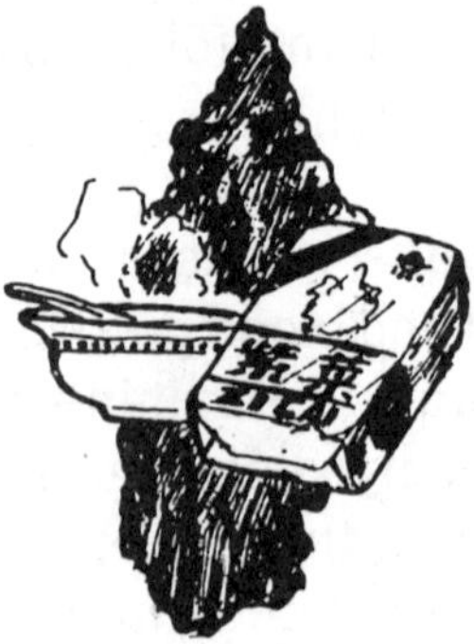

16. Laver

A plant belonging to red alga now cultivated artificially on a large scale.

Nature and flavour: Sweet, salty and moderate.

Constituents: Containing protein, fat, sugar, cellulose, carrotene, vitamins B_1, B_2 and C, iodine, calcium, phosphorus and iron.

Pharmacology: Disaggregating and softening actions.

Indications: For simple goitre, tuberculous lymphadenitis and chronic bronchitis.

B. Roots and Stems

1. Ginger

A plant belonging to the zingiberacea family. There are two kinds of ginger, the tender and the old. For medicinal use the latter is mostly applied.

Nature and flavour: Pungent and warm (the tender ginger is slightly warm).

Constituents: Its main content is zingetone which is hot, and composed of zingiberol, zingiberene, camphene, citral, etc.

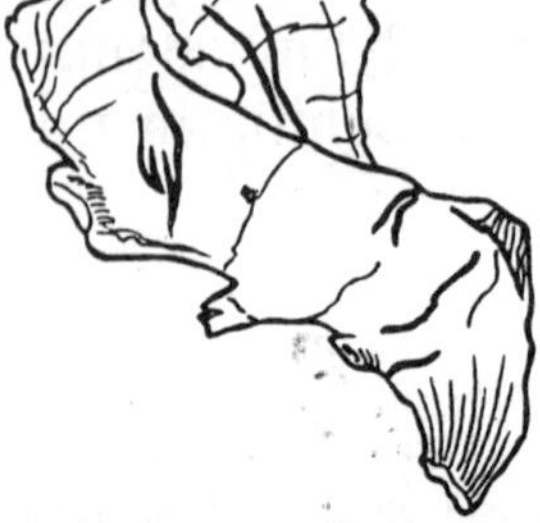

Pharmacology: It has the actions of stimulating the central nervous system, diaphoresis, stopping vomiting and detoxifying. It also stimulates blood circulation and strengthens stomach function.

Indications: Flu of the evil-wind cold type and all kinds of vomiting. For chronic bronchitis in the elderly, mix half a teaspoonful of ginger juice with syrup and swallow with hot water.

2. Lily

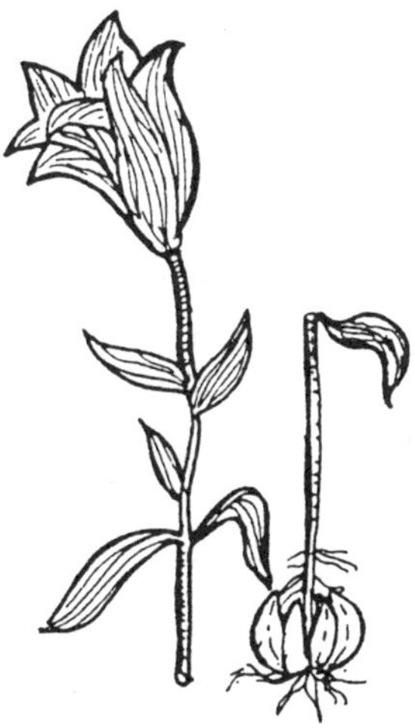

A plant belonging to the lily family. Both natural and domestic species serve for medicinal purposes. The bulbs are the part used.

Nature and flavour: Sweet and moderate.

Constituents: Containing protein, fat, several alkaloids and a considerable amount of starch. Calcium, phosphorus and iron are also present.

Pharmacology: Antitussive and anti-asthmatic action.

Indications: Stopping coughs, moistening the lungs, with benefiting and nourishing actions. Applied for pulmonary tuberculosis, emphysema and chronic bronchitis.

3. Sweet potato

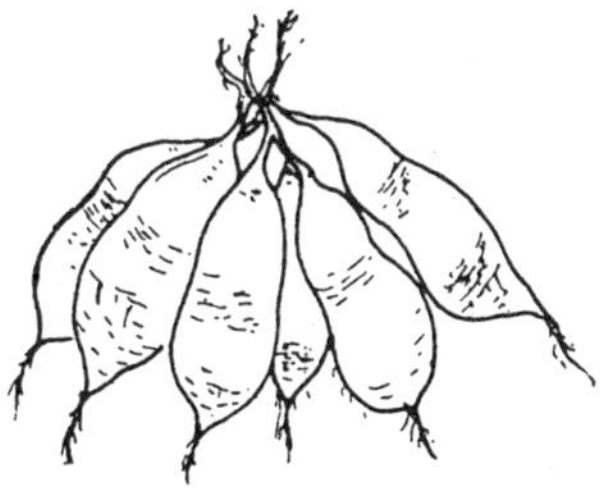

A plant belonging to the convolulacea family.

Nature and flavour: Sweet and moderate.

Constituents: Large amounts of starch, carrotene, cellulose and mucin.

Indications: Strengthening the spleen and stomach, benefiting the vital energy. Good for poor digestion. It is also effective for night blindness, best taken with animal liver.

4. Potato

A plant belonging to the solanacea family. Its underground stem is the edible portion, the skin of which may be white, yellow or purple in colour.

Nature and flavour: Sweet and moderate.

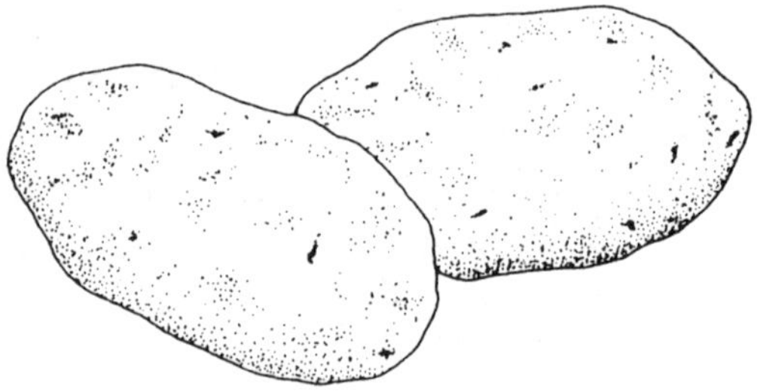

Constituents: Containing large amounts of starch, protein, colloid material, vitamins B_1 and C, and potassium. Also containing solanin.

Pharmacology: Solanin possesses the action of relieving gastrointestinal tract spasms and decreases the secretions of the stomach.

Indications: Regulating the functions of the spleen and stomach. Mostly applied for gastric and duodenal ulcers. Mix its juice with honey and take before breakfast. Also applied externally for skin eczema.

Note: Potatoes sprouted should not be eaten.

5. Water chestnut

The underground bulb of a plant belonging to the Cyperacea family.

Nature and flavour: Sweet and cold.

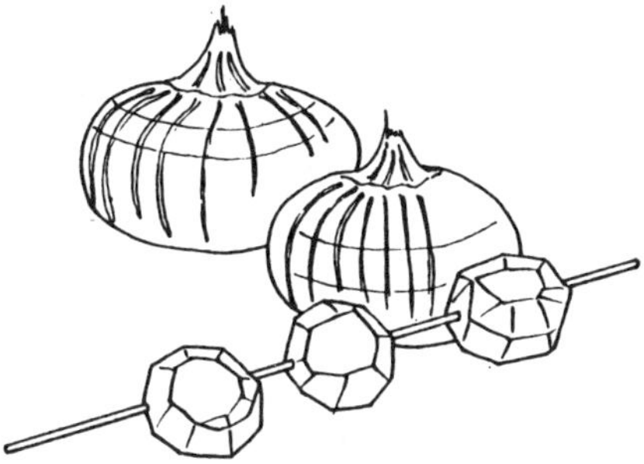

Constituents: Containing rich starch and also fat and protein, vitamin C, calcium, phosphorus and iron.

Pharmacology: The puchiin contained in water chestnut reveals an inhibitory action on Bacillus coli and Staphylococcus aureous.

Indications: Hypertension, chronic bronchitis, coughing.

6. Polygonum multiflorum (the tuber of multiflower knotweed)

Belonging to the polygonacea family. The tubers are mainly used, though its stem, termed *yejiaoteng*, is also used as a medicine.

Nature and flavour: Bitter, slightly warm.

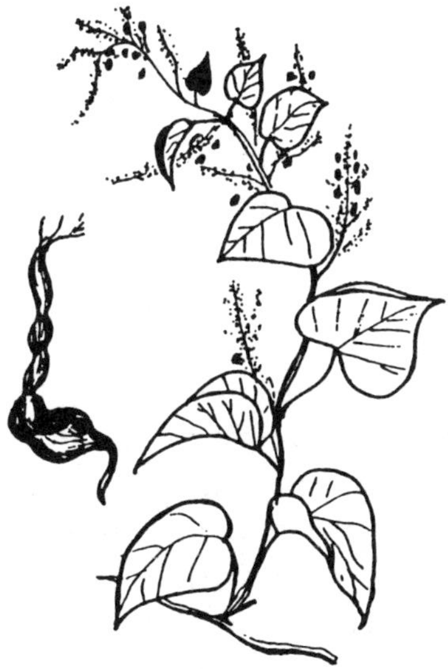

Constituents: Containing chrysophanol, emodin, rhein, and chrysophanic acid, and anthrone.

Pharmacology: In animal experiments the extract of its tuber stimulates the locomotion of the intestines, and promotes the functions of digestion and absorption. It also lowers blood fats and blood sugar.

Indications: Used as subsidiary treatment for hypertension and arteriosclerosis. In traditional

Chinese medicine, it is claimed to tonify blood and vital energy, and blacken hair.

7. Taro

A plant belonging to the aracea family with a variety of species. Its bulb stem is edible and the raw taro is used for medical purposes.

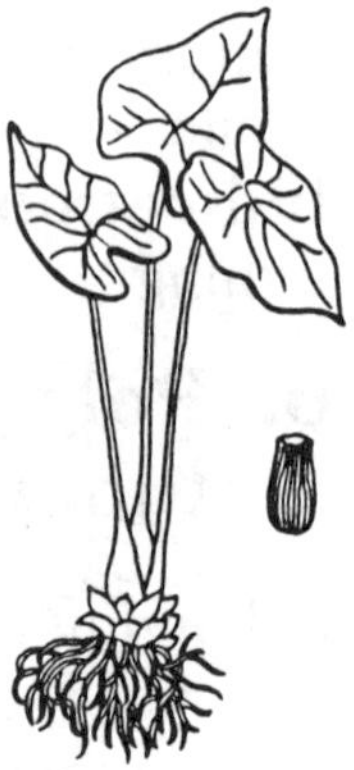

Nature and flavour: Pungent and moderate. Raw taro is slightly toxic.

Constituents: Containing protein, fat, starch, calcium, phosphorus and iron. Also containing mucin, saponin, carrotene, and vitamins B_1, B_2 and C.

Pharmacology: It has the action of nourishing the spleen and stomach, and anti-inflammation and analgesic actions.

Indications: Swelling of lymph nodes, tuberculous lymphadenitis. External use for boils and carbuncles, ulcers and mastitis.

8. Alli macrostem's bulb

A plant belonging to the liliacea family. Its tuber root is used for medicinal and dietary purposes. Since its root is white in colour, hence the name white *xie* in Chinese.

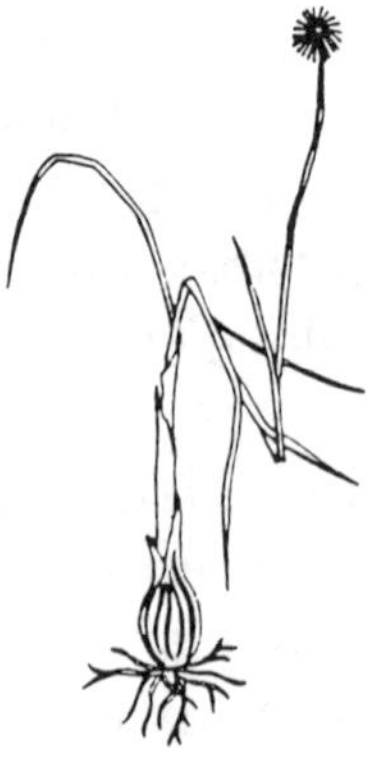

Nature and flavour: Bitter, pungent and warm.

Constituents: Consisting mainly of allicin.

Indications: For dispersing stagnation and depression, warming the interior. Chest distress and angina due to coronary diseases can be treated by this bulb, associated with Chinese trichosanthes (snakegourd fruit). Also good for dysentery.

9. Chinese yam

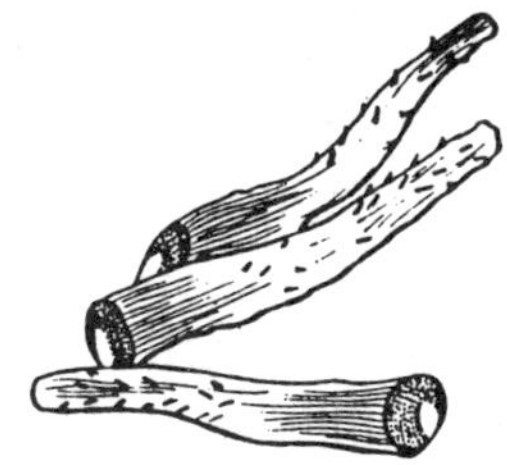

A plant belonging to the dioscoreacea family. Its tuber root is used for medicinal purposes.

Nature and flavour: Sweet and moderate.

Constituents: Containing saponin, mucin, choline, glycoprotein, free amino acid, abscisin, etc. Also rich in starch and vitamin C.

Action: It is a nourishing agent, promoting digestion, producing body fluids and stopping thirst.

Indications: Diabetes mellitus, chronic diarrhoea due to deficiency of the spleen function.

10. Turnip

A plant belonging to the crucifera family, including a great variety of species, such as those with white skin, red skin, green skin with red flesh (called *xinlimei* in northern China), long shape, oval shape, etc. However, their therapeutic usage is basically the same. The tuber root and seeds are all used for medical purposes; the red skin and white skin species are most commonly used.

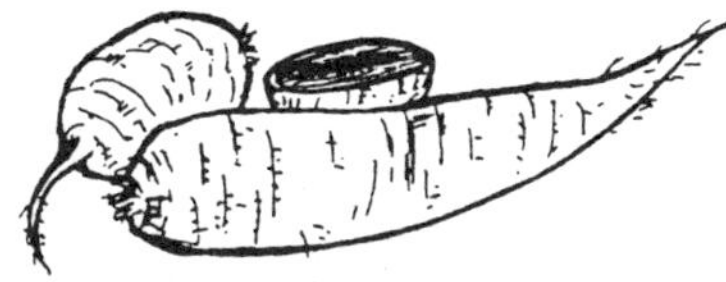

Nature and flavour: Sweet, pungent and slightly cool.

Constituents: The tuber root contains affluent water with glucose, sucrose and fructose. In addition there is also caffeic acid, ferulic acid, benzo-pyruvic acid and many kinds of amino acid. Fresh turnip also contains vitamin C, calcium, manganese and boron. In the seeds there is volatile oil, fatty acid and raphanusin.

Pharmacology: Extracts from tuber root of turnip have anti-bacterial action, so do the seeds. In traditional Chinese medicine, it is claimed that turnip promotes digestion, strengthens the spleen, and has antitussive, antipyretic and detoxication actions.

Indications: Bronchitis, laryngitis, common cold and dyspepsia.

11. Carrot

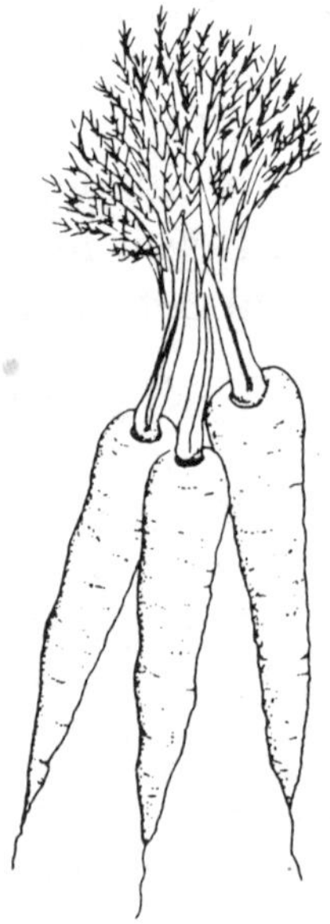

A plant belonging to the umbellifera family. Its seeds are also used for medicinal purposes.

Nature and flavour: Sweet and slightly warm.

Constituents: Rich in carrotene, sugar, fatty acid, volatile oil and umbelliferone.

Pharmacology: In animal experiments, its extract reveals the action of lowering blood sugar.

Indications: Night blindness. Best taken fresh. The wild species shows helminthagogue action.

12. Wild rice stem

A marine plant belonging to the graminea family. Its tender and thick stem serves as a medicine.

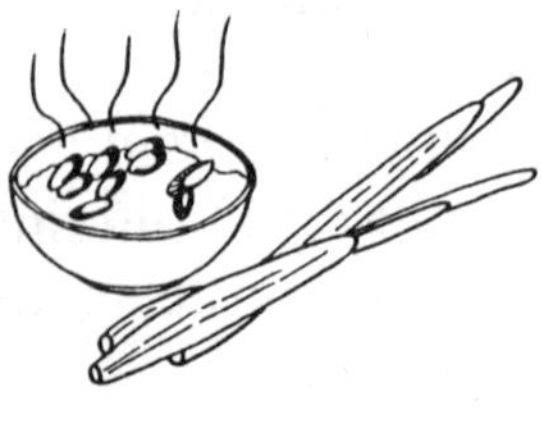

Nature and flavour: Sweet and cold.

Constituents: Containing fat, protein and cellulose.

Indications: It has the actions of diuresis and relieving thirst and is administered for hypertension and lack of milk secretion after delivery.

13. Sugar cane

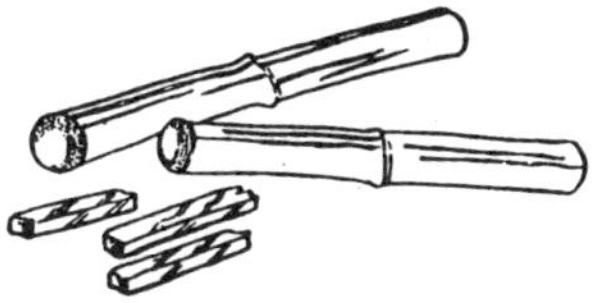

A plant belonging to the graminea family. Its stem is used for medical purposes.

Nature and flavour: Sweet, moderate and slightly cold.

Constituents: Containing affluent water, and sugar, fat, protein, calcium, phosphorus and iron.

Indications: It reveals actions of strengthening digestive functions, relieving thirst and eliminating sputum, and is administered for coughing, vomiting and nausea due to heat of deficiency type.

14. Lotus root

Lotus root is a plant belonging to the nymphaeacea family. All its parts are used for medicinal purposes.

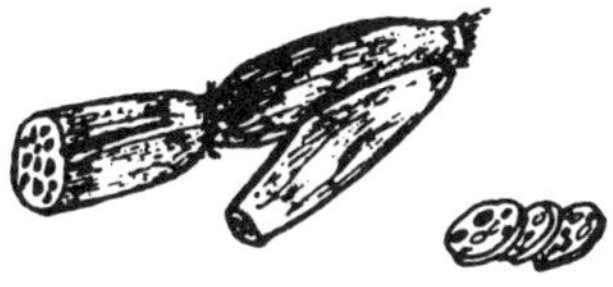

Nature and flavour: Sweet, moderate and slightly cold.

Constituents: The root is rich in starch, tannate and vitamins B and C.

The stem contains alkaloid, resin and tannate. The seeds are rich in asparagin, fat, protein and starch, and the leaves are rich in nuciferine, nornuciferine, roemerine and quarcetin.

Action: Lotus seeds are nourishing and sedative, the leaves, the pod of the seeds and stem are hemostatic and astringent, while the root is a conventional hemostatic agent.

Indications: For all kinds of bleeding including hemoptysis hematemesis, nose bleeding, vaginal, uterine bleeding, hematochezia. For chronic diarrhoea use lotus stem decoction. For haemophilia, use fresh root.

15. Onion

A very common plant belonging to the liliacea family. Its bulb stem is used for medicinal purposes.

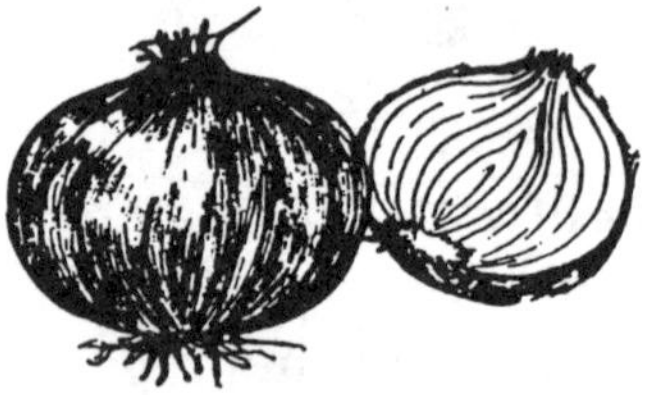

Constituents: Rather complicated. Containing thiol, quercetin, ferulic acid and many amino acids.

Action: Bactericidal. Promoting gastric secretion. Also an antiseptic for trichomonas vaginalis.

Indications: For non-bacterial dysenteric diarrhoea, use one to two onions and serve as a common dish at meals.

C. Flowers, Seeds, Gourds and Fruits

1. Osmanthus flower

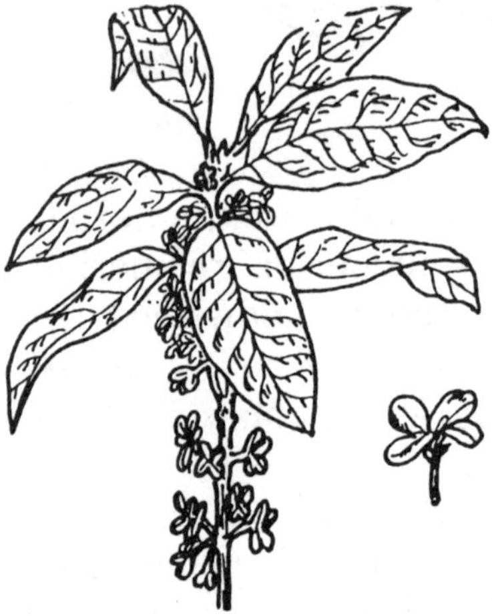

A flower of the osmanthus belonging to the oleacea family. It has a very strong fragrance.

Nature and flavour: Sweet, pungent and slightly warm.

Constituents: Volatile oil, geraniol.

Action: Warming the interior and eliminating evil cold, stopping pain and warming the stomach.

Indications: Stomach pains due to evil cold, belching and abdominal distention.

2. Chrysanthemum

There are many varieties of chrysanthemum, of which only some species are used for medicinal purposes. It is mainly made into a tea-like drink.

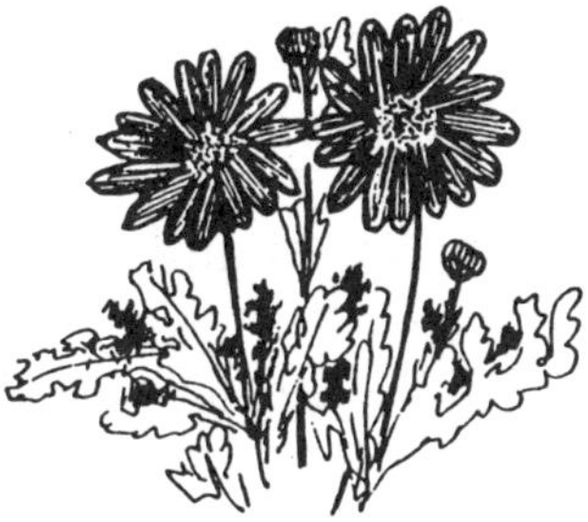

Nature and flavour: Bitter, sweet and moderate.

Constituents: Chrysanthemum, adenine, amino acids, choline, stachydrine, etc.

Pharmacology: It has the anti-bacterial action and strengthens the tenacity of capillary vessels.

Action: In traditional Chinese medicine, it is claimed that chrysanthemum clears fever and eliminates evil dampness, relieves dizziness and improves eye-sight.

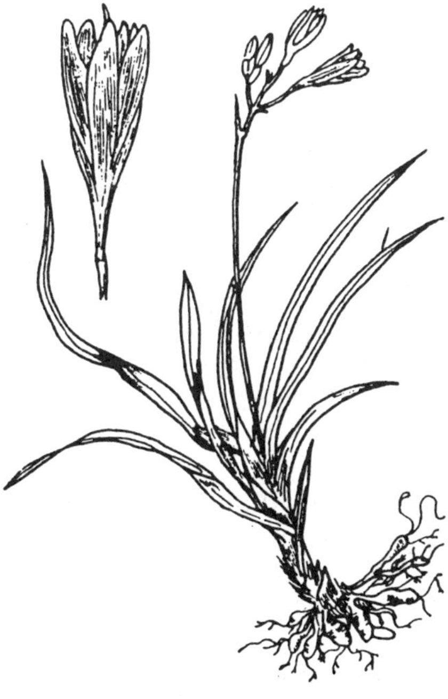

3. Day lily

In China, it is also called yellow-flower vegetable and belongs to the liliacea family.

Nature and flavour: Sweet and cool.

Constituents: Containing asparagin,

colchicine, vitamins A, B, and C, protein and anthraquinone A, B, C, D and F.

Action: Anti-inflammation, antipyretic and analgesic. Also having diuretic action and relieving deep-coloured urine in children.

Indications: Infectious hepatitis, bleeding (hematemesis, hemoptysis and epistaxis), and mastitis.

4. Tomato

A plant belonging to the solanacea family with special odour.

Nature and flavour: Sour, slightly sweet and moderate.

Constituents: Containing large amounts of water, vitamins C, B_1 and B_2, calcium, phosphorus, iron, carrotene and a small quantity of tomatine.

Pharmacology: The alkaline contained in the fruit is effective on many bacteria and fungi. In animal experiments, tomato juice shows the actions of lowering blood pressure and stimulating the smooth muscle. In traditional Chinese medicine, it is claimed that the tomato bears antipyretic and detoxifying actions.

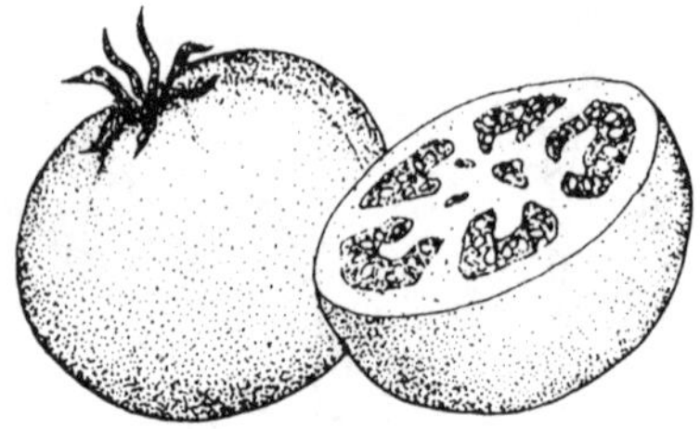

Indications: For some effect on hypertension, take 1-2 tomatoes every morning before breakfast.

5. Peanut

A plant belonging to the leguminosa family.

Nature and flavour: Sweet and moderate.

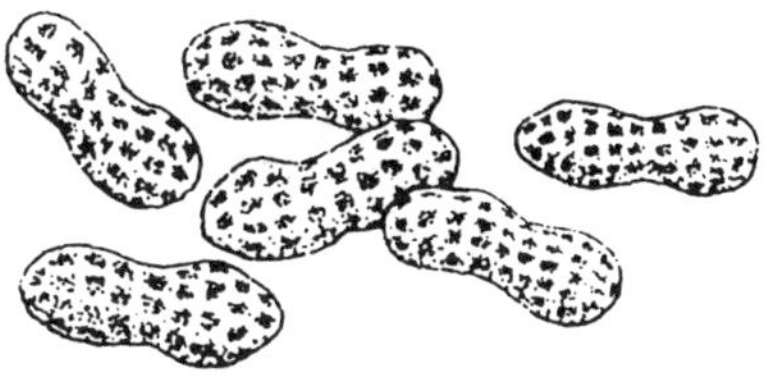

Constituents: Containing large amounts of fat, also vitamins A, B, E, and K, lecithin, choline, amino acids, calcium, etc.

Pharmacology: Experiments show that peanut with its membranous skin shortens coagulation time. Peanut oil lowers blood pressure and blood cholesterol. The membrane contains even more effective ingredients.

Indications: Haemophilia, epistaxis, purpura, chronic nephritis, leukorrhagia and insomnia.

6. Red bean

A plant belonging to the leguminosa family. The whole bean is red in colour and is easy to distinguish from the jequirity bean which, though similar in shape, is half red and half black and is toxic.

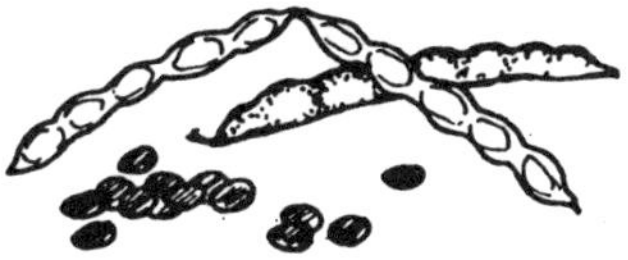

Nature and flavour: Sweet and moderate.

Constituents: Containing starch, protein and fat, vitamins A, B and C, saponin, aluminium and copper.

Action: Diuretic, antiphlogistic and detoxifying.

Indications: Effective for nephritis, beriberi, malnutrition, and edema. Also effective for erysipelas and other carbuncles.

7. Hyacinth bean

A plant belonging to the leguminosa family.

Nature and flavour: Sweet and slightly warm.

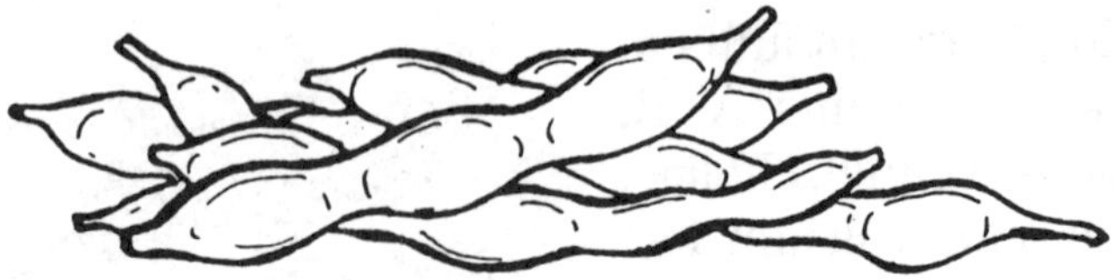

Constituents: Containing protein, fat and sugar. Also with panthothenic acid, calcium, phosphorus, iron, zinc and magnesium.

Action: Strengthening the spleen and stomach, eliminating evil dampness and summer heat, anti-diarrhoea.

Indications: Diarrhoea due to summer heat. Also for vomiting and diarrhoea in acute gastro-enteritis. Thirst in heat-stroke and leukorrhagia, rheumatic arthritis.

8. Cowpea

A plant belonging to the leguminosa family.

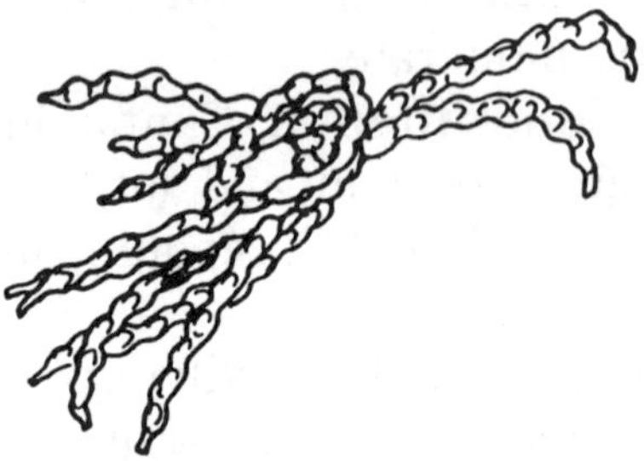

Nature and flavour: Sweet, salty and moderate.

Constituents: Containing starch, fat and protein. Also containing nicotinic acid, vitamins B_1 and B_2.

Action: Strengthening the spleen, regulating digestive function, benefiting vital energy and relieving thirst.

Indications: Diabetes mellitus, thirst and polyuria.

9. Broad bean

A plant belonging to the leguminosa family.

Nature and flavour: Sweet, slightly pungent and moderate.

Constituents: Containing protein, fat and carbohydrate, amino acid, vitamins B_1 and B_2.

Action: Hemostatic action. Its skin is a diuretic and relieves edema.

Indications: Hypertension, hemoptysis, epistaxis and leukorrhagia.

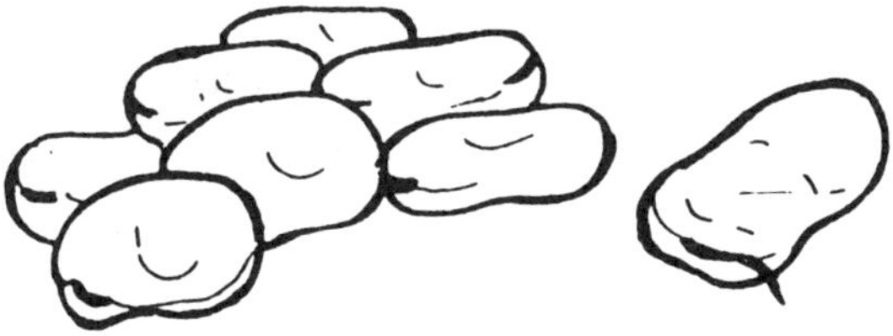

Note: Children who reveal fever and jaundice after eating broad beans, especially the fresh raw ones, should be sent to a hospital or clinic immediately.

10. Black bean

A plant belonging to the leguminosa family. Its wild species called *Maliao* bean is best for medicinal uses.

Nature and flavour: Sweet and moderate.

Constituents: Containing fat, protein and sugar, vitamin B_1, nicotinic acid and melanin.

Action: Diuretic and detoxicant. Its skin has nourishing and anti-perspiration actions.

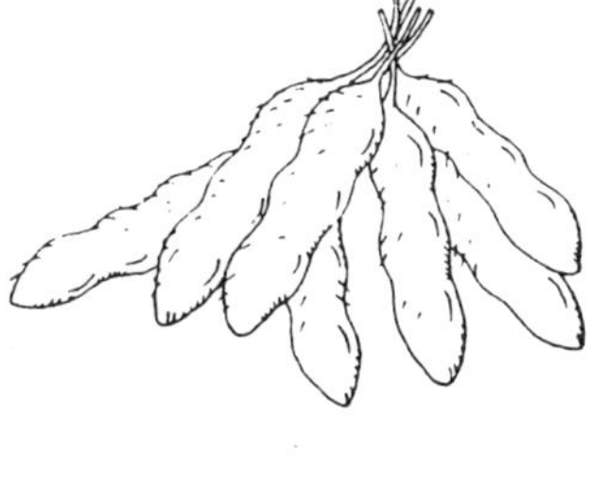

Indications: Common cold, night sweating, spontaneous sweating, weakness after severe illness, postpartum rheumatic pains.

11. Green bean

A plant belonging to the leguminosa family.

Nature and flavour: Sweet and cold.

Constituents: Containing protein, fat, starch, vitamins A, B_1, and B_2, calcium, phosphorus and iron.

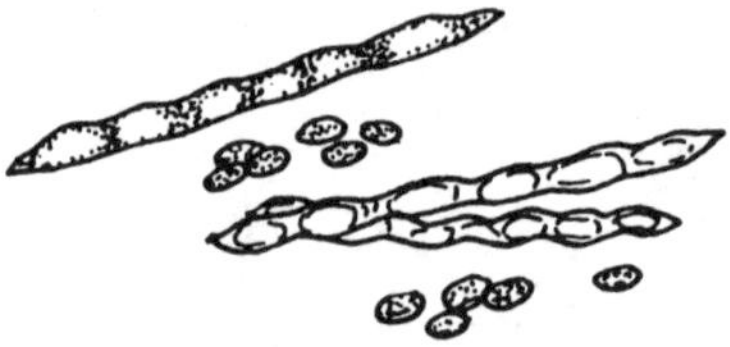

Action: Diuretic and relieving swelling, antipyretic, detoxifying, cooling and good for summer heat.

Indications: Summer heat, especially good in the hottest summer days. In food poisoning, it detoxifies. It is also applied for preventing heat stroke and cures eczema and boils by local application.

12. Soybean

A plant belonging to the leguminosa family.

Nature and flavour: Sweet, moderate and slightly cold.

Constituents: Containing large amounts of protein (40 percent), hence the name "vegetable meat". Also

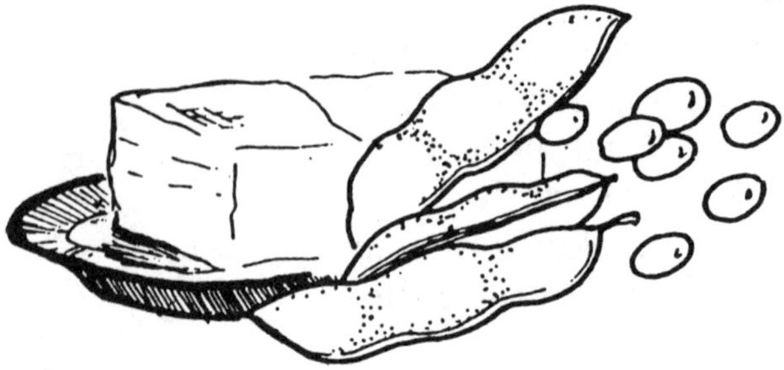

containing fat, iron, calcium, carrotene and vitamins B_1 and B_2.

Action: Activating blood, detoxification and diuretic action.

Indications: Common cold, diarrhoea (bake the bean skin until scorched and grind into powder, administer orally). For boils when applied locally.

13. Palm starch grain

This grain is made from the starch prepared from the medulle of Metroxylong sagu Rottb, a plant belonging to the palm family.

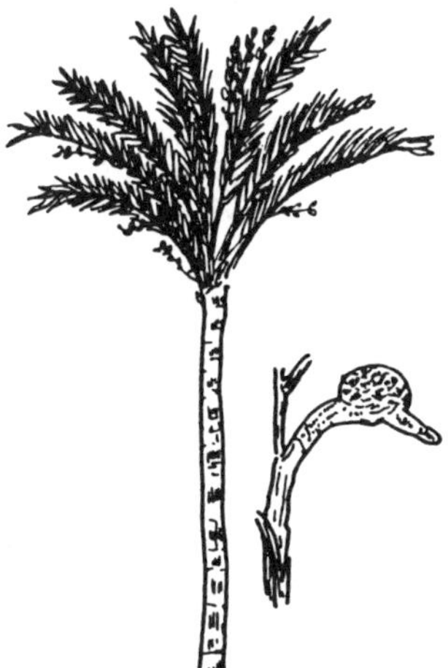

Nature and flavour: Sweet, moderate and warm.

Constituents: Mainly composed of starch.

Action: Strengthening the spleen, warming the interior, benefiting the lungs and eliminating sputum.

Indications: Deficiency of the spleen-stomach functions, dyspepsia of deficient-cold type. Weakness due to severe illness or postpartum.

14. Husked sorghum

A grain belonging to the graminea family.

Nature and flavour: Sweet and slightly cold.

Constituents: Mainly composed of fat, protein, starch and protosugar.

Action: Effective for insomnia coupled with dyspepsia due to weakness of the spleen-stomach functions.

Indications: Mainly postpartum weakness, insomnia and general weakness.

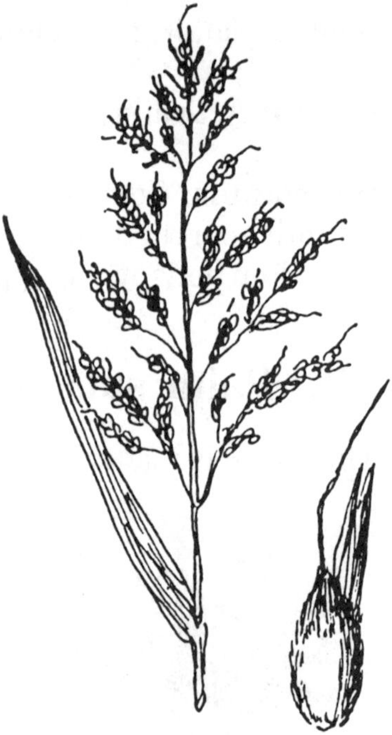

15. Maize

A plant belonging to the graminea family.

Nature and flavour: Sweet and moderate.

Constituents: Mainly fatty acid, volatile oil, resin, zeaxanthin, saponin, alkaloids. The seeds contain protein, vitamins B_1, B_2 and B_6, calcium, phosphorus and iron.

Pharmacology: It may lower blood pressure and blood sugar, hemostatic. Its diuretic action is extrarenal in nature.

Indications: Diabetes, urinary stone, urgency of micturition, polyuria, pain during urination, acute and chronic cystitis, edema due to nephritis.

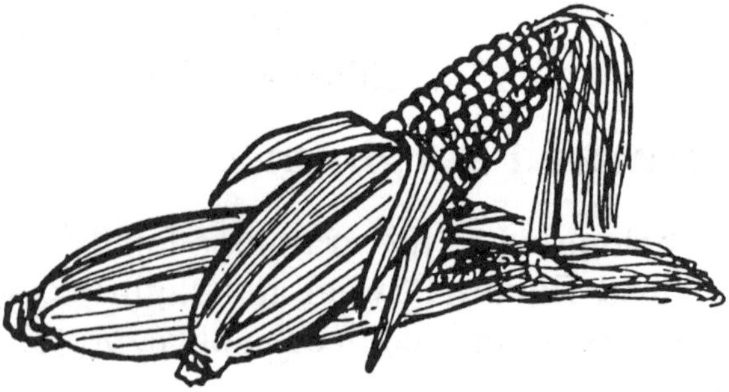

16. Wheat

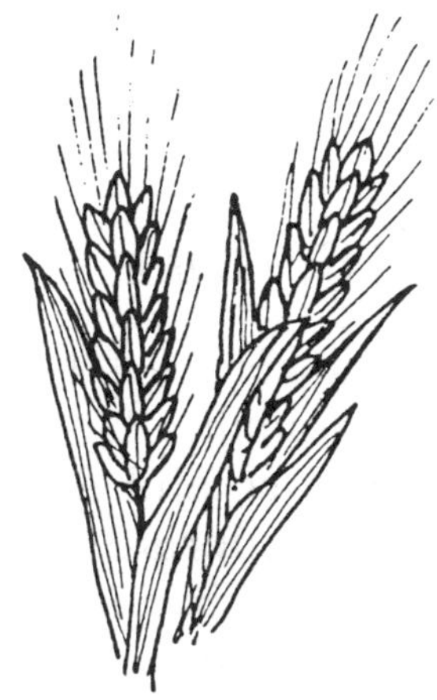

A plant belonging to the graminea family, the staple food in North China. Floating wheat refers to those dry and shrivelled grains which float on the surface of water.

Nature and flavour: Sweet and slightly cold.

Constituents: Containing protein, starch, saccharin, fat, cellulose, ergosteroid, lecithin, allantoin, amylase and vitamin B.

Action: Beneficial to the heart and mind, relieving perspiration due to asthenia.

Indications: Idiopathic perspiration, palpitation, night sweating, and hysteria (in association with administration of glycyrrhiza and dates).

17. Barley

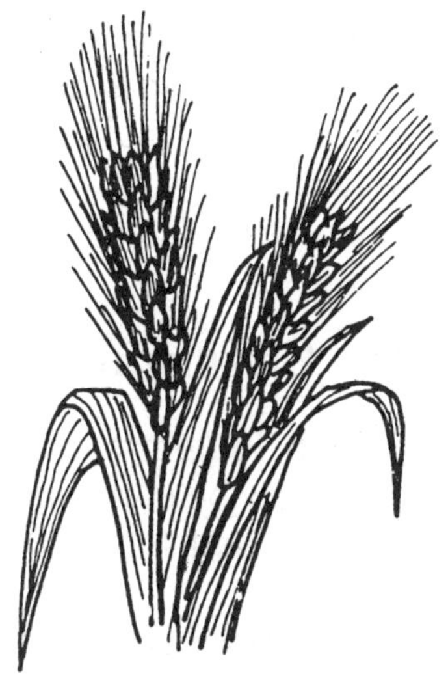

A plant belonging to the graminea family. Its sprout is used for medicinal purposes.

Nature and flavour: Salty and warm.

Constituents: Containing maltose, glucose, saccharin, lecithin, amylase and vitamin B.

Action: Benefiting the functions of the spleen and stomach, and relieving dyspepsia.

Indications: Dyspepsia, weakness in digestion, especially in children, weakness as a sequala of hepatitis, inducing interruption of lactating secretion for mothers.

18. Rice

The kernel of the seeds of the plant rice, belonging to the graminea family. It may be husked or unhusked.

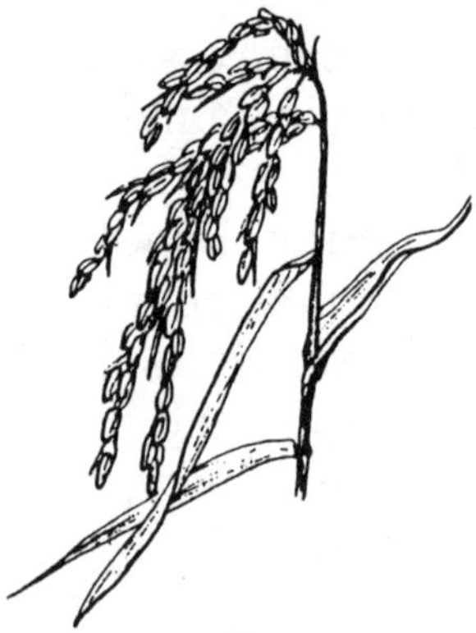

Nature and flavour: Sweet and moderate (warm when produced in northern China).

Constituents: Rich in starch with a little protein and some vitamin B.

Action: Beneficial to the functions of the spleen and stomach.

Indications: Rice should be boiled at a low heat until it is sticky. For medicinal purposes, poria and fruit of Chinese wolfberry may also be added to reinforce its nourishing actions.

19. Chestnut

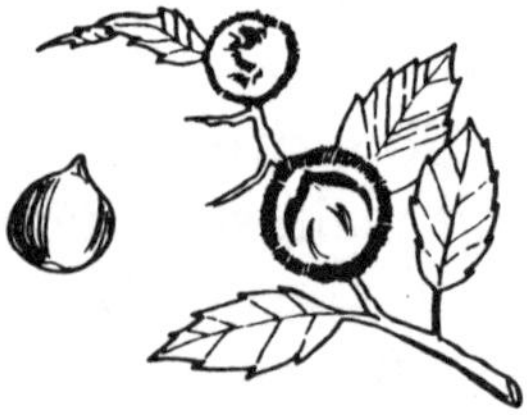

A plant belonging to the fagacea family. It may be domestic or wild. Its fruit is used for medical purposes.

Nature and flavour: Sweet and warm.

Constituents: Rich in starch and sugar, protein, fat, and vitamins B_1 and B_2.

Action: Nourishing the spleen and stomach, and benefiting the vital energy.

Indications: Weakness of spleen-stomach functions in the elderly, frequent urination and infantile diarrhoea. Several raw pieces may be chewed for treatment.

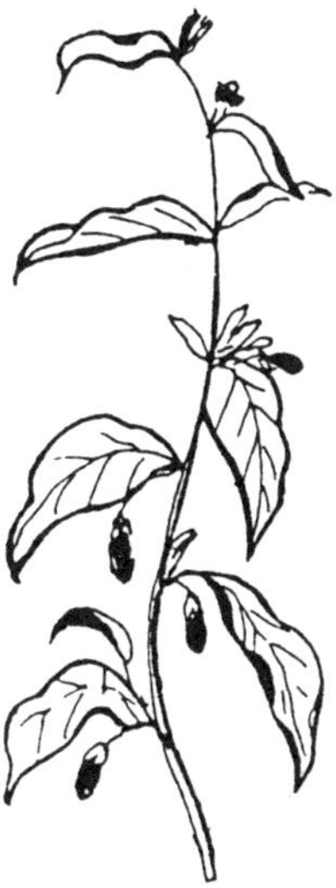

20. Fruit of Chinese wolfberry

A plant belonging to the solanacea family. Its tender leaves are edible and the fruit is used as a medicinal food.

Nature and flavour: Sweet and moderate.

Constituents: Containing carrotene, vitamins B_1, B_2 and C, β-ergosteroid and lenoleic acid.

Pharmacology: It possesses an antagonistic action to fatty depositions in the liver and lowers blood sugar. In traditional Chinese medicine, it is claimed that this fruit improves eye-sight, nourishes vital essence, benefits the kidney and stomach and is a diuretic.

Indications: Hypertension, diabetes mellitus, night blindness, dizziness and seminal emissions due to weakened kidneys.

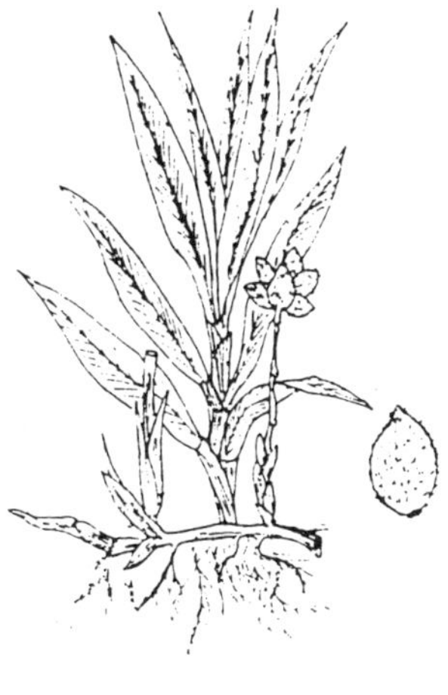

21. Fructus amomi

An aromatic flavouring produced from a plant belonging to the zingiberacea family.

Nature and flavour: Pungent and warm.

Constituents: Volatile oil, camphor, bornyl acetate, d-Borneol, linalool, etc.

Action: Stomachic, regulating the circulation of vital energy in the body, warming up the spleen and kidney. Relieving vomiting and dyspepsia.

Indications: Weakness of the spleen and stomach. Dyspepsia of cold-deficient type. Hematemesis and diarrhoea of watery stool.

22. Pepper

There are two kinds of pepper, black and white both belonging to the piperacea family.

Nature and flavour: Pungent and hot.

Constituents: Containing piperine, chavicine, piperanine, cryptone, caryophyllene oxide, etc.

Pharmacology: Expelling evil-wind, strengthening stomach action, and serving as an antipyretic for certain kinds of cold.

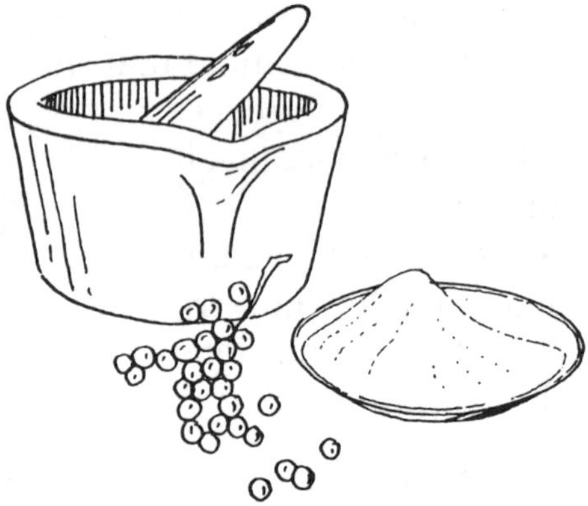

Indications: Abdominal pains of a cold and deficient type, common cold of evil wind-cold type. Nausea and vomiting.

23. Chilli

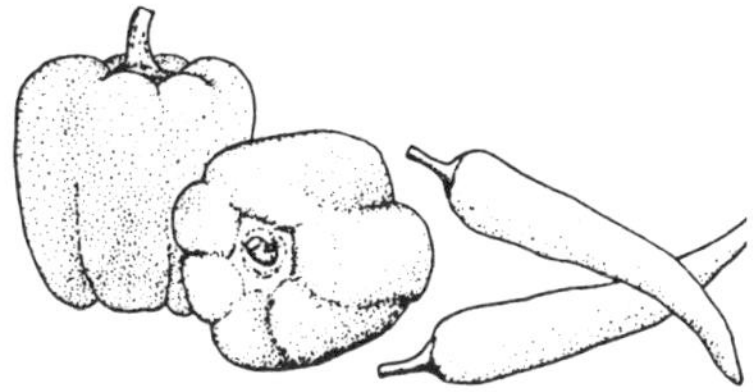

A plant belonging to the solanacea family, with a great variety of species different in shape and with different quantities of chilli elements.

Nature and flavour: Pungent and warm.

Constituents: Capsaicin, capsanthin, fatty oil, solanidine, solanine and considerable amount of vitamin C.

Pharmacology: It stimulates appetite, stimulates the digestive tract, increasing its blood volume and promoting circulation, and also shows inhibitory action on bacillus subtilis.

Action: Increasing the secretion of digestive fluids. Also effective for deficiency of digestive function.

Indications: Weakness of digestive function (cold type). Its lotion is effective for frostbite and baldness when applied by local washing.

Note: Contraindicated to peptic ulcer patients.

24. Chinese prickly ash

A plant belonging to the rutacea family.

Nature and flavour: Pungent and warm.

Constituents: Volatile oil, limonene, cumic alcohol, geraniol, steriod and unsaturated organic acid.

Pharmacology: It has extensive inhibitory action on bacteria, among others streptococcus hemolyticus, diphtheria, dysentery, typhoid fever bacilli and pseudomonas aeruginosa. It also promotes the growth of some glands (such as gonads).

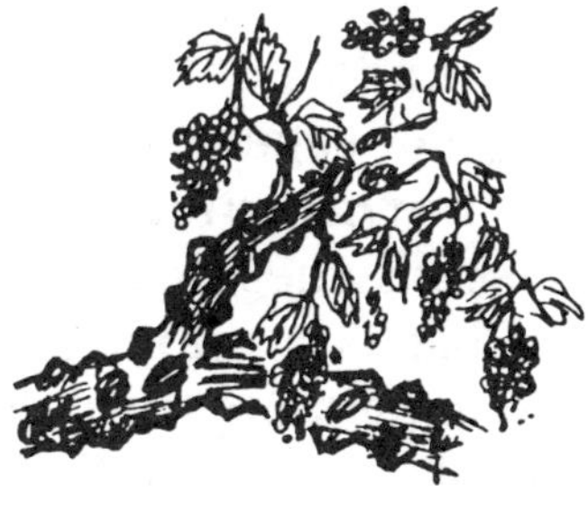

Indications: Rheumatism of joints and muscles, chronic nephritis, abdominal pains due to ascaris.

25. Aniseed

A plant belonging to the magnoliacea family.

Nature and flavour: Pungent and moderate.

Constituents: Volatile oil, fatty acid, protein and resin.

Pharmacology: Its alcohol extract inhibits the growth of some bacteria in vitro. In traditional Chinese medicine, it is claimed that aniseed warms the interior, stops pain, cures evil coldness in the abdomen and stops vomiting.

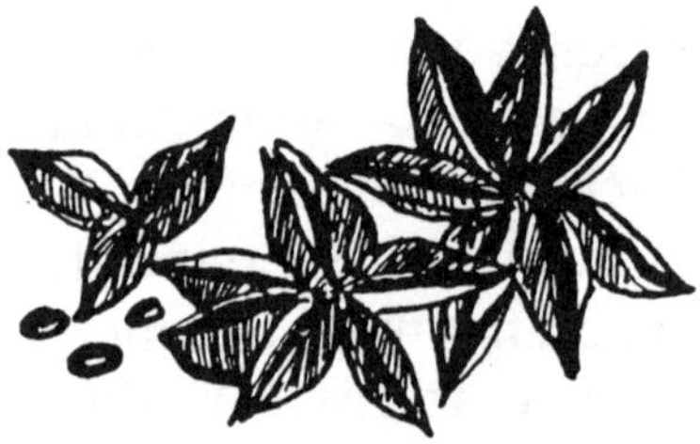

Indications: Pain in lower abdomen, abdominal distention, constipation, scantiness and redness of urine due to hernia.

26. Clove

A tropical plant belonging to the myrtacea family.

Nature and flavour: Pungent and warm.

Constituents: Clove oil in the buds contains mainly eugenol, eugenin and chavicol.

Pharmacology: It possesses some inhibitory effect on bacteria. Stomachic and stopping toothache. In traditional Chinese medicine, it is

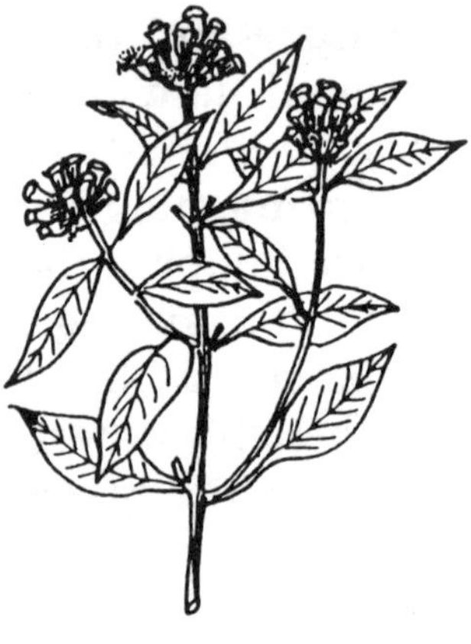

claimed that it warms the spleen and stomach and stops vomiting.

Indications: Vomiting and hiccup due to evil coldness of stomach.

27. Olive

The fruit of a plant belonging to the burseracea family.

Nature and flavour: Sweet, sour and warm.

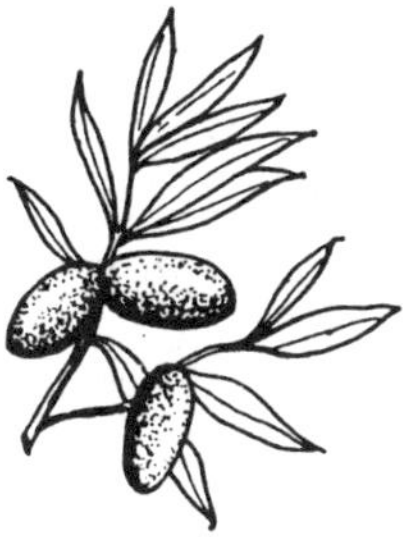

Constituents: It contains protein, fat, sugar, vitamin C, calcium, phosphorus and iron.

Action: Nourishing body fluids and detoxification, eliminating sputum and good for sore throat.

Indications: For sore throat due to upper respiratory infection, and abdominal pain due to toxification by some fish, crabs and globefish. Also applied for fishbone stuck in the pharynx.

28. Sunflower

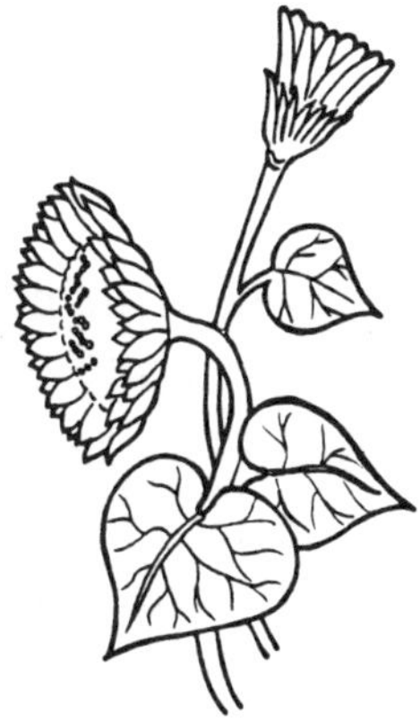

A plant belonging to the composita family. Its seed dish, flower, and stem are all used for medicinal purposes.

Nature and flavour: Sweet and moderate.

Constituents: The oil from its seeds contains glyceride and linolenic acid, glyceride. Its stem contains polysaccharide and chlorogenic acid.

Pharmacology: Animal experiments reveal that the oil from its seeds prevents hyperlipemia and hypercholesterolemia. Extracts from the flower and the dish prevent hypertension. In traditional Chinese medicine, it is claimed to subdue endogenous wind due to excessive function of liver, and eliminates evil heat.

Indications: Headache and dizziness due to hypertension, abdominal pain during menstruation and asthma. The flower disc can also be used for treatment.

29. Seed of Job's tear

The seed from a plant belonging to the graminea family.

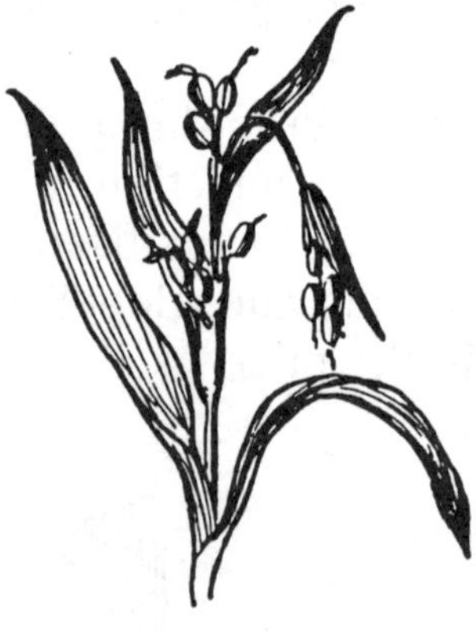

Nature and flavour: Sweet and slightly cold.

Constituents: Sugar, fat, protein, coixol, coixenolide and triterpenes.

Action: Benefiting the spleen functions, eliminating edema, diuretic and nourishing the digestive functions. In animal experiments it shows some anti-cancer effect.

Indications: For dyspepsia, cystitis, urethritis with deep coloured urine, urodynia and frequent urination. Furthermore, its root is good for jaundice and oliguria.

30. Hawthorn

The fruit of a plant belonging to the rosacea family with various species.

Nature and flavour: Sweet, sour and slightly warm.

Constituents: Protein, fat, rich in vitamin C, hawthorn acid, lemon acid, saponin, tannate and fructose.

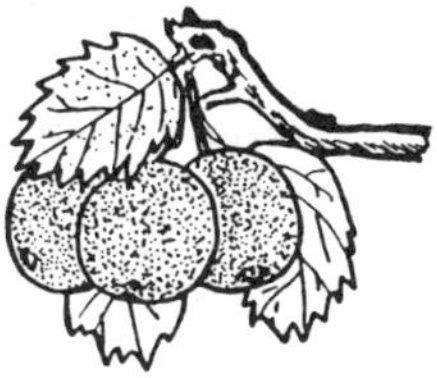

Pharmacology: Increasing secretion of digestive juices, especially beneficial for the digestion of meat. Anti-bacterial, softening the blood vessels and lowering blood pressure and blood cholesterol. In traditional Chinese medicine, it is held that it cures dyspepsia and emaciation in children, and eliminates vomiting, pain and diarrhoea.

Indications: For indigestion due to eating too much meat, dyspepsia, coronary heart disease, hypertension, scurvy, post-partum abdominal pains due to blood stagnation, diarrhoea, etc.

31. Sesame

Belonging to the pedaliacea family. There are two kinds of sesame, black and white.

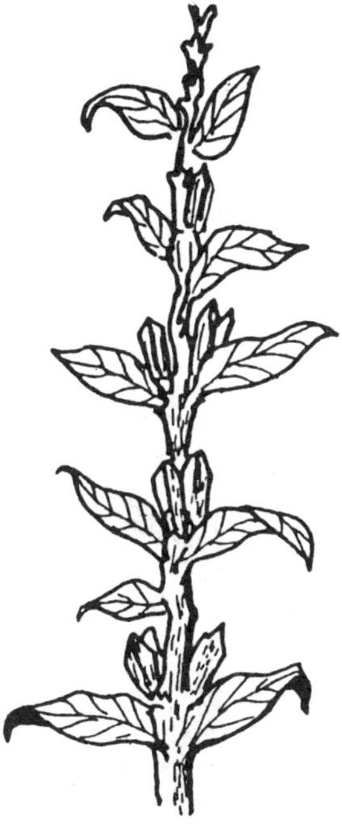

Nature and flavour: Sweet and moderate.

Constituents: It contains much fat, mainly glyceride of oleic acid and loneleic acid, sucrose, lecithin, protein, sesamine, sesamol, etc.

Action: Strengthening the body, lubricating for defecation, beneficial to the liver and spleen and blackening the hair.

Indications: Mainly for blood deficiency and deficiency of vital essence (yin), constipation, dry and white hair, coughing and short breath in the elderly. Chronic pharyngitis.

32. Eggplant

A plant belonging to the solanacea family. There are many kinds of eggplant, elongated and oval shape, white and purplish skin, etc.

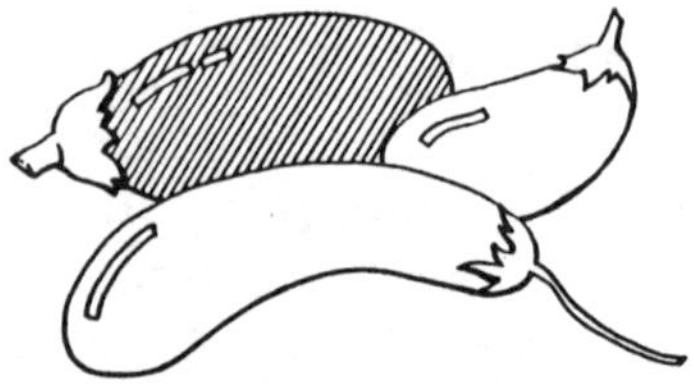

Nature and flavour: Sweet and cold.

Constituents: It contains trigonelline, stachydrine, choline, solanine, vitamins B and C, nicotinic acid, carrotene, protein and fat.

Action: Astringent, activating blood, analgesic, hemostatic, diuretic and detoxifying.

Indications: Chronic bronchitis, rheumatic arthritis, leukorrhagia. Also good for frostbite, toothache and metroptosis when applied locally.

33. Calabash

A plant belonging to the cucurbitacea family. The species with the narrow-waisted fruit is applied for medical use.

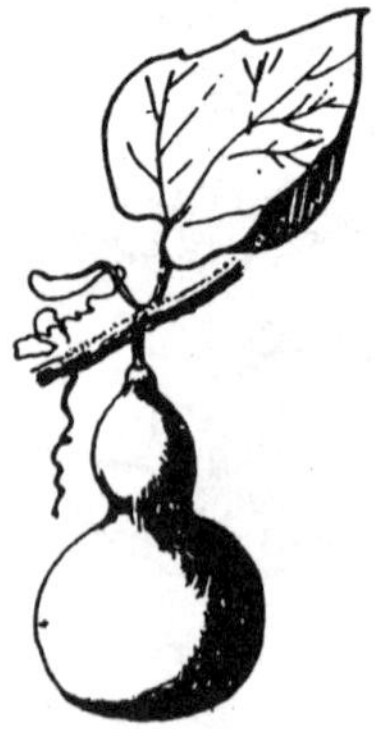

Nature and flavour: Sweet and moderate.

Constituents: The flesh in dry calabash contains glucose. Raw calabash contains carrotene, vitamins B and C, protein and fat.

Action: With marked diuretic action. For distension of the abdomen and edema.

Indications: Cardiac and hepatic edema, oliguria, thirst and feverish sensations in hypertension.

34. White gourd

A plant belonging to the cucurbitacea family. Its skin and seeds are used for medicinal purposes. The flesh is also used.

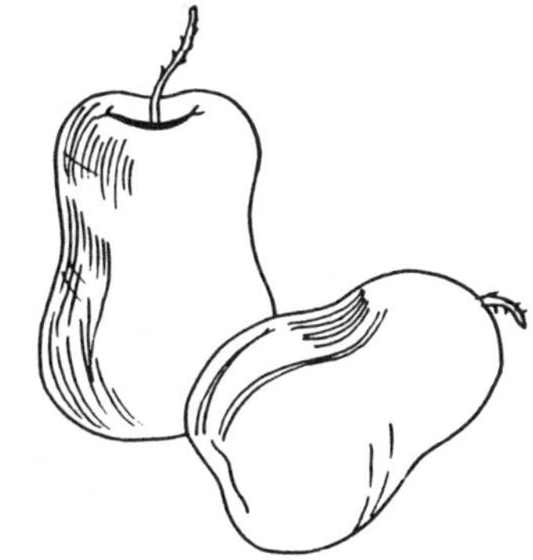

Nature and flavour: Sweet and slightly cold.

Constituents: Mostly water, with some sugar, protein, cellulose, carrotene, vitamins B, B_1 and B_2, calcium, phosphorus and iron.

Action: Marked diuretic action, especially the skin portion of the plant. The seeds are good for ulcers of the viscera as an antiphlogistic.

Indications: Thirst in heatstroke, cardiac and hepatic edema, oliguria. It may be used as subsidiary therapy for lung and intestinal ulcers.

35. Pumpkin

A plant belonging to the cucurbitacea family.

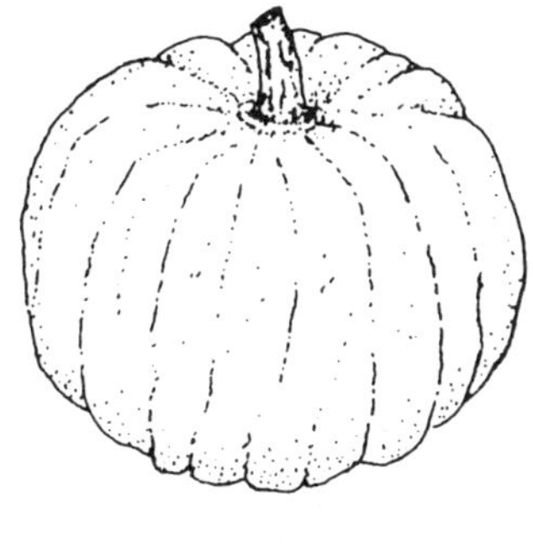

Nature and flavour: Sweet and cold.

Constituents: It contains trigonelline, adenine, carrotene, vitamins B and C, glucose and sucrose. The seeds contain fat and protein.

Action: The flesh is beneficial to spleen functions, whereas the seeds are anthelminthic. It is antiphlogistic and analgesic when applied locally.

Indications: For elimination of tape worm, fasciolopsiasis and schistosomiasis, chronic bronchitis, ascites and oliguria.

36. Water-melon

The fruit of a plant belonging to the cucurbitacea family. It is good for overcoming summer heat.

Nature and flavour: Sweet and cold.

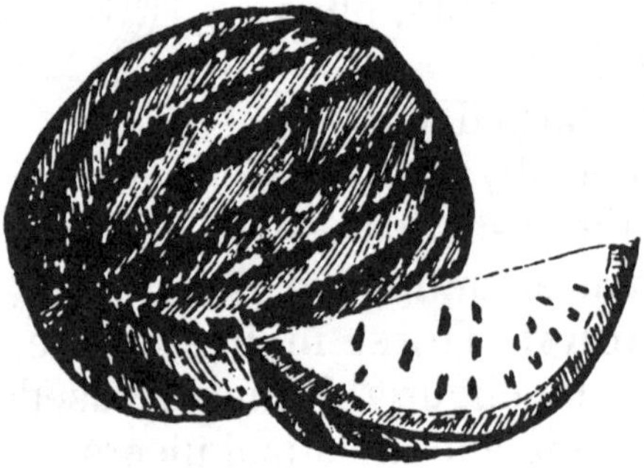

Constituents: The flesh contains phosphoric acid, malic acid, fructose, glucose, amino acid, lycopene, carrotene and vitamin C. The seeds contain fat and vitamin B_2.

Action: Eliminating summer heat thirst, and diuresis.

Indications: Hypertension, heatstroke, acute and chronic nephritis, pharygo laryngitis, edema, etc.

37. Dark plum

The fruit of a plant belonging to the rosacea family. Made by smoking unripe green plum.

Nature and flavour: Sour and moderate.

Constituents: It contains malic acid, citric acid, succinic acid, β-sitosterol, triterpene, etc.

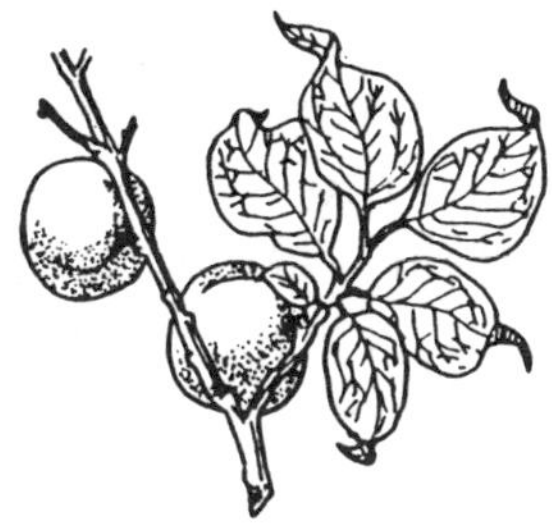

Pharmacology: Marked antibacterical action, especially to bacillus E coli, dysentery, typhoid fever, cholera bacilli and Pseudomonas aeruginosa. In traditional Chinese medicine, it is an antipyretic, antiascaris remedy with astringent action.

Indications: Effective on typhoid, paratyphoid fever, biliary ascariasis, etc.

38. Chinese date (including wild jujube)

There are many kinds of dates in China, including red, black and wild jujube, all belonging to the rhamnacea family.

Nature and flavour: Red dates are sweet and moderate, wild jujube sour and moderate.

Constituents: Protein, sugar, organic acid, and mucus. Rich in vitamins B_2, C, and P.

Action: It possesses the action of relieving and nourishing, while wild jujube's seeds are a sedative.

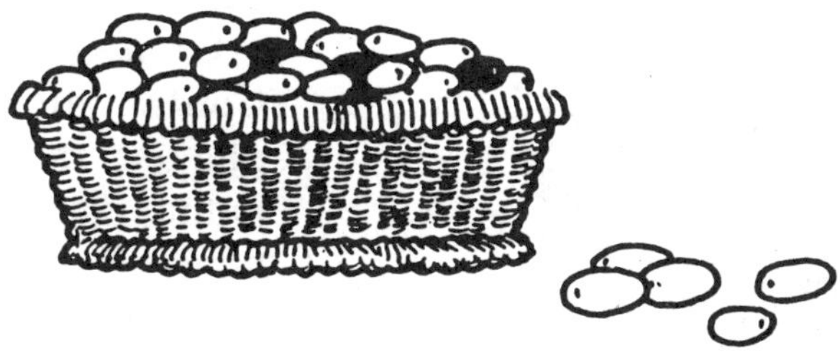

Indications: Anaphylactic purpura, abdominal pains due to enteritis, urticaria, and sweating due to weakness. Wild jujube's seeds are mostly used for insomnia and neurasthenia.

39. Pear

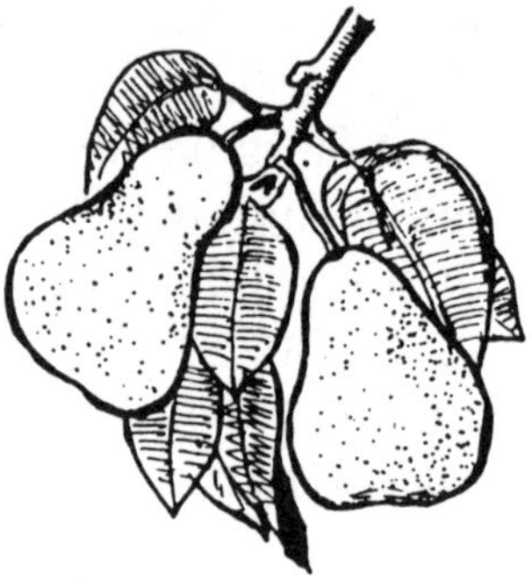

The fruit of a plant belonging to the rosacea family, including various species. For medicinal use, those with thin skin, tender and juicy flesh are preferable.

Nature and flavour: Sweet and cold.

Constituents: Containing malic acid, glucose, sucrose, vitamins B and C.

Action: Moistening the lungs, elimination of sputum, antipyretic and antitussive actions.

Indications: Acute and chronic bronchitis, coughing with sputum or without sputum, hard to cough up.

40. Persimmon

The fruit of a plant belonging to the ebenacea family. Both fresh and dried persimmon are used for medicinal purposes.

Nature and flavour: Sweet and cold. The white powder on the surface of dried persimmon is sweet and moderate, while the calyx is puckery.

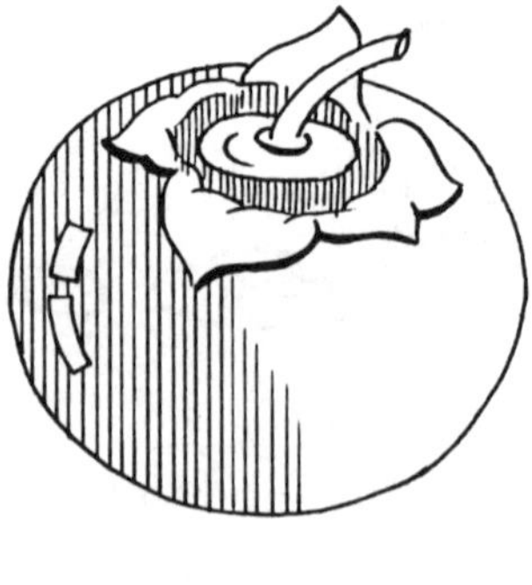

Constituents: Containing sucrose, glucose, fructose and iodine. The calyx contains triterpene, olive acid and ursolic acid. Powder of dried persimmon contains manitole, glucose, fructose, sucrose and vitamin C.

Pharmacology: The astragalin extracted from persimmon leaves lowers blood pressure and increases blood flow in coronary arteries. In TCM*, it is claimed that persimmon is an antipyretic, while its dry white powder moistens the lungs and heart. The calyx is good for hiccup. Persimmon is capable of lowering blood pressure and is good for constipation.

Indications: Hypertension, chronic bronchitis, and hiccup.

41. Loquat

A plant belonging to the rosacea family. The fruit, kernel and tender leaves are all used for medicinal purposes.

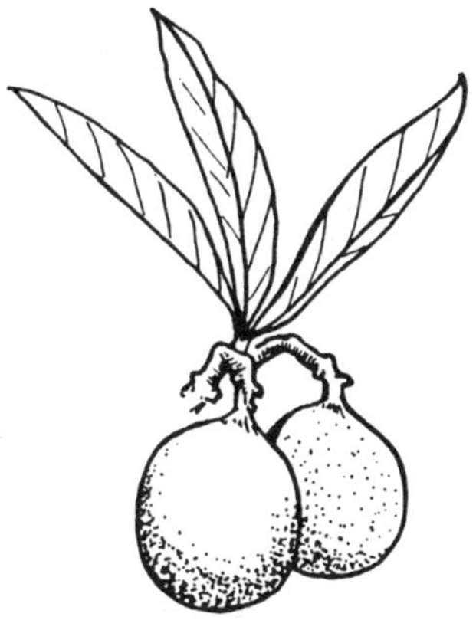

Nature and flavour: Sweet, sour and moderate.

Constituents: Its flesh contains malic acid, tartaric acid, citric acid, tannate, carrotene, vitamins A, B and C. Its leaves and kernel contain anygdalin.

Action: Beneficial to the vital energy of the lungs. Relieving coughing and vomiting. The flesh promotes the secretion of body fluids and eliminates thirst. The tender leaves, free of hairs, are antitussive and eliminate sputum.

Indications: Coughing due to evil heat in the lungs. Chronic and acute bronchitis. Thirst due to evil summer heat can be treated with loquat leaves, drunk as a substitute for tea.

*Traditional Chinese Medicine

42. Tangerine

The fruit of a plant belonging to the rutacea family. The species vary. Besides its flesh, the skin and pith are also used for medicinal purposes.

Nature and flavour: Flesh (sweet, sour and warm). Skin (pungent and warm).

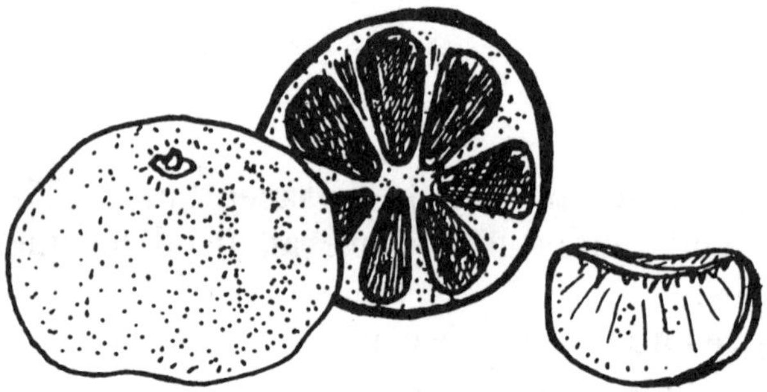

Constituents: Hesperidin, citric acid and citrene. Its flesh contains malic acid, citric acid and sucrose, with a large quantity of vitamin C and carrotene.

Action: Tangerine skin regulates the vital energy, stops cough, eliminates sputum and invigorates functioning of the stomach. Its pith is beneficial to the lungs and clearing the channels.

Indications: When associated with other medicines, it cures vomiting and coughing due to cold of the lungs in flu and acute bronchitis.

43. Banana

The fruit of a plant belonging to the musacea family.

Nature and flavour: Sweet and cold.

Constituents: It contains starch, protein, fat, vitamins A, B, C and E and a little nor-adrenaline.

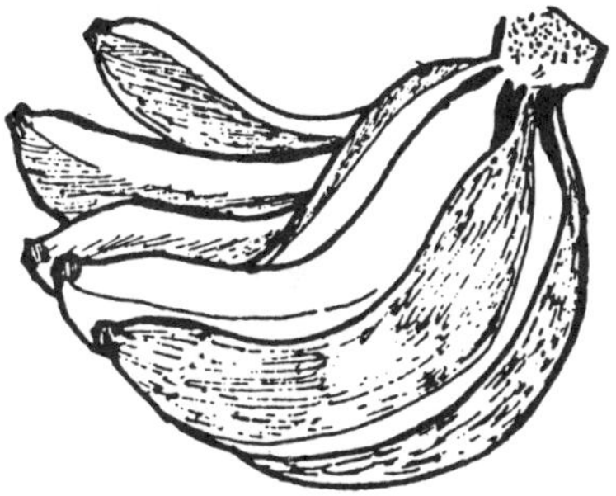

Action: A lubricant for defecation. Also an inhibition to fungus and bacteria and a blood pressure lowering agent.

Indications: Disturbance of digestive function (take 2-3 once). Banana flowers bear some action on preventing encephlorrhagia.

44. Pomegranate

The fruit of a plant belonging to the punicacea family. The skin is used for medicinal purposes.

Nature and flavour: Sweet, sour and warm.

Constituents: The fruit skin contains tannic acid, resin, innosital, sugar, and gum. The skin of its root contains isopelletierine.

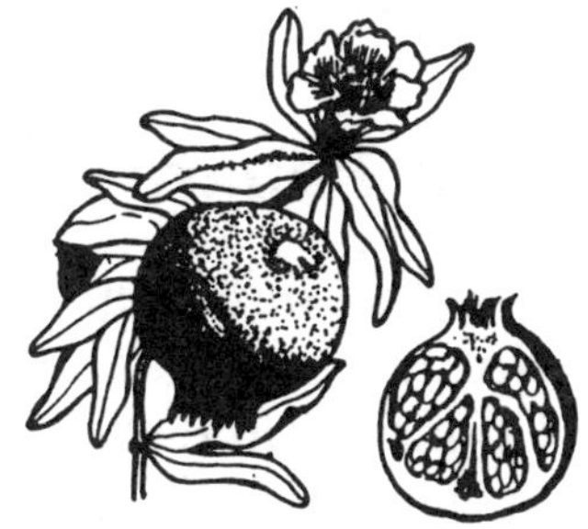

Pharmacology: The skin of its root is an anthelminthic. Pomegranate skin reveals strong inhibition to typhoid bacilli. In TCM, it is an astringent.

Indications: Chronic diarrhoea, including dysentery and enteritis. Also for tape worm and ascaris.

45. Almond

The fruit of a plant belonging to the rosacea family. There are two kinds of almond, bitter and sweet.

Nature and flavour: Sweet and warm, or bitter and warm.

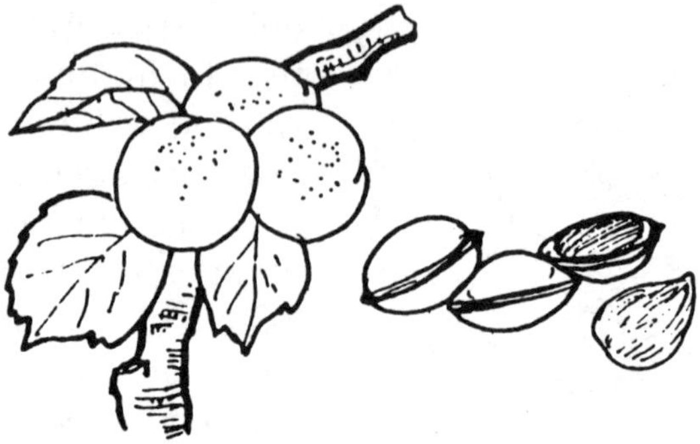

Constituents: Sweet almond contains amygdalin, fat, sugar, protein, resin, mandelnitrite, and apricot oil; and bitter almond contains amygdalin and fat.

Action: Bitter almond is best for antitussive and anti-asthmatic action, while sweet almond is mostly applied for the weak and elderly for antitussive purposes.

Indications: Chronic bronchitis, coughing and asthma in the elderly.

46. Papaya

The fruit of a plant belonging to the caricacea family.

Nature and flavour: Sweet and cold.

Constituents: Rich in sugar, also containing organic acid, fat, protein, vitamins B and C. In matured fruit, there are sticky and milky secretions with fat-enzyme (lipase) and protein enzyme.

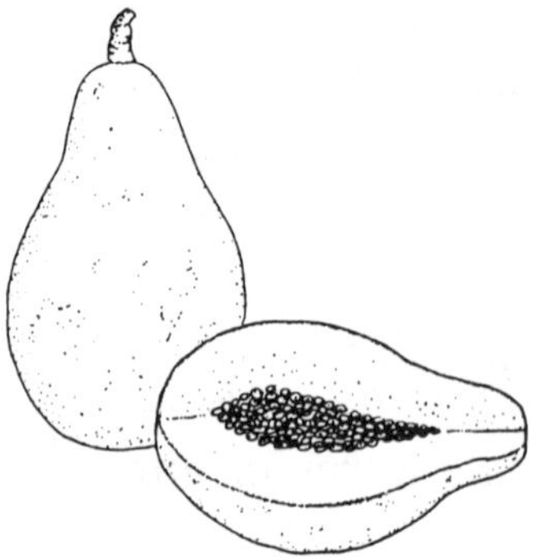

Pharmacology: Aside from being beneficial to digestion, it is also helpful to the dissolution of fat, having body-strengthening, digestion-improving and anti-cancer actions, as well as eliminating summer heat and thirst.

Indications: Chronic dyspepsia and anti-tapeworm. Also for boils and carbuncles when applied locally.

47. Gingko

Commonly called "silver-apricot", it belongs to the ginkgoasea family. Its fruit is used for medicinal purposes.

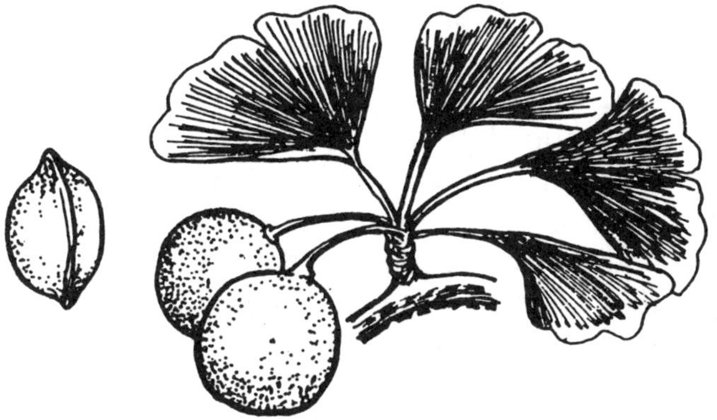

Nature and flavour: Sweet, bitter, puckery and toxic.

Constituents: Containing ginkgolic acid, sugar, tannate, fatty oil, starch and protein.

Action: Beneficial to the vital energy of the lungs and anti-asthmatic.

Indications: Bronchial asthma (10-12 g boiled in water and administered as a decoction with residue. It may be also administered after baking). The raw fruit can be applied locally for boils and ulcers.

Note: Gingko is toxic and should not be administered in excessive amounts, as this would produce vomiting, fever or even convulsions.

48. Walnut

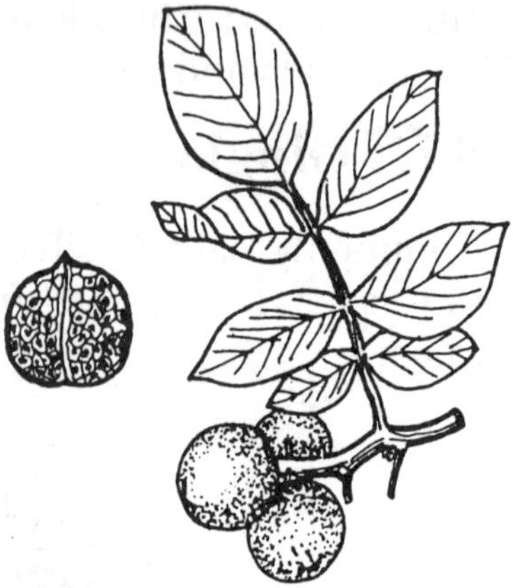

The fruit of a plant belonging to the jugladacea family.

Nature and flavour: Sweet and warm.

Constituents: Containing much fat, also protein, vitamins B_1 and B_2, tannate and juglone.

Action: The fat in walnut is beneficial to the formation of albumin in the body. In TCM, it is claimed that walnut is warm yet not dry like most nuts; hence, it is good for weakness and deficient vital essence in the elderly, nourishing the blood and vital energy, benefiting the lungs and kidney and moistening the lungs.

Indications: Chronic bronchitis with coughing and asthma in the elderly, polyuria due to kidney deficiency, senile habitual constipation or diarrhoea, etc.

49. Mulberry fruit

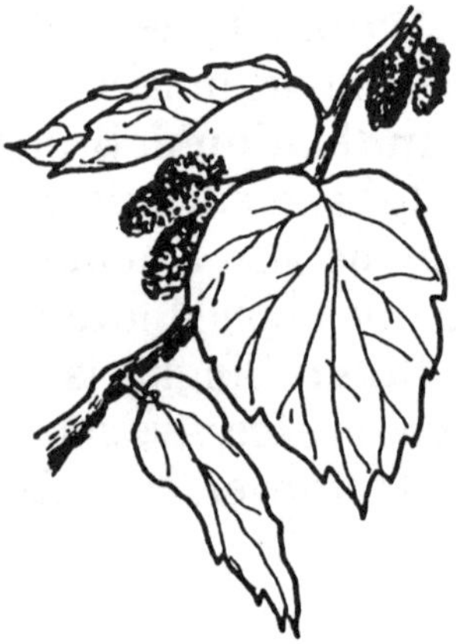

The fruit of a plant belonging to the moracea family.

Nature and flavour: Sweet and moderate.

Constituents: Rich in carrotene, vitamins B_1, B_2 and C, glucose, sucrose, tartaric acid and succinic acid.

Action: Benefiting vital energy and eliminating excessive fluids.

Indications: Rheumatic arthritis, numbness, pain, anaemia and neurasthenia.

50. Dried longan pulp

The fruit of a plant belonging to the sapindacea family. The dried fruit is used for medicinal purposes.

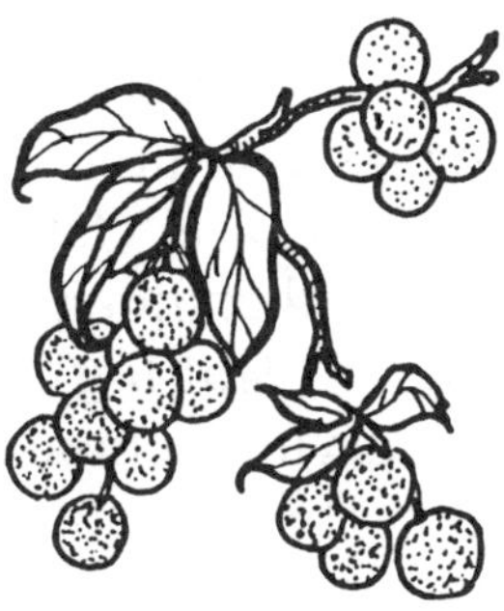

Nature and flavour: Sweet and warm.

Constituents: Rich in glucose and vitamin B, tartaric acid, protein and fat.

Action: Beneficial to the spleen and heart; a blood tonic with its kernel having astringent and hemostatic actions.

Indications: Anaemia, neurasthenia, spontaneous sweating, night seating, insomnia and palpitations.

Note: Since it is a warm fruit, do not take too much at a time.

51. Grape

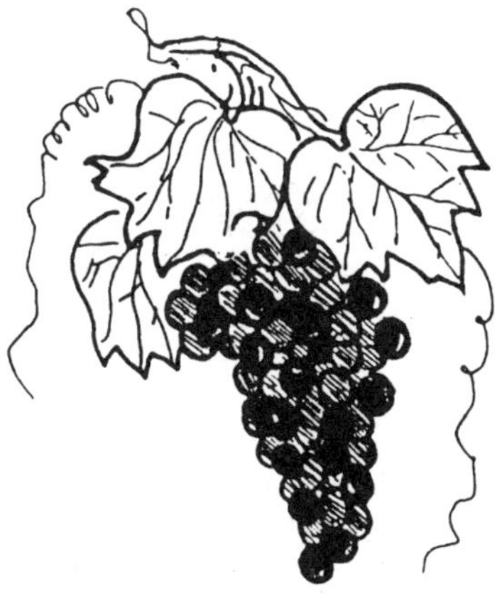

The fruit of a plant belonging to the vitacea family. It is, together with its wine, highly nutritious.

Nature and flavour: Sweet and moderate.

Constituents: Containing polysaccharides, protein, vitamins B_1, B_2 and C.

Action: After fermenting into wine, it is a strong blood tonic.

Indications: Weakness and anaemia. Take a small amount every day. Too much wine is harmful.

52. Guava

The fruit of a plant belonging to the myrtacea family.

Nature and flavour: Sweet and moderate.

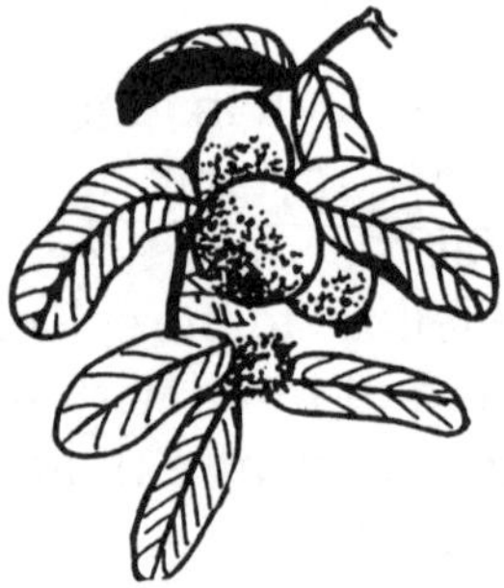

Constituents: The fruit contains β-sitosterol, guaijaverin, vitamin C, sugars and quercetin.

Action: In TCM, it is claimed that guava stops diarrhoea and bleeding, with antiphlogistic, astringent and drying actions.

Indications: The fruit juice is a remedy for diabetes mellitus. The green and immature fruit, after having been baked and ground into powder, is good for wounds.

53. Bitter gourd

A plant belonging to the cucurbitacea family.

Nature and flavour: Bitter and cold.

Constituents: Containing charantin, 5-hydroxytryptamine, vitamin C, etc.

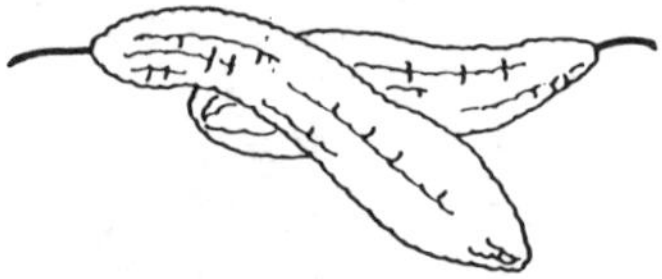

Action: It is claimed, in TCM, that this gourd clears the evil fire of the heart and improves eyesight, while its fruit strengthens the vital energy and sexual power.

Indications: For boils, and erysipelas on the leg due to summer heat, take it as food, while the leaves, after grinding, can be applied locally. The seeds, after baking and grinding into powder, are good for impotence.

54. Carambola

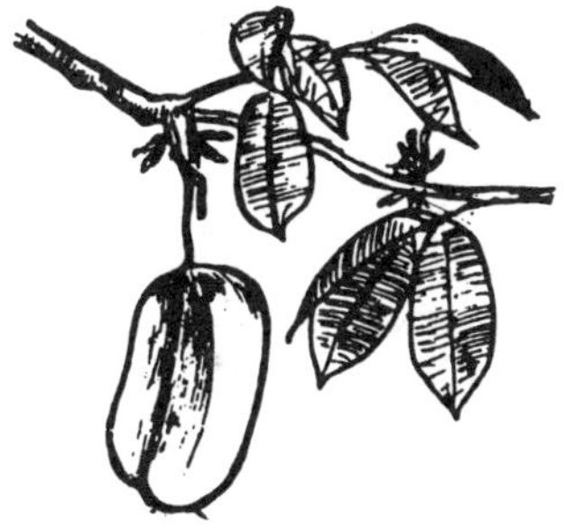

The fruit of a plant belonging to the cucurbitacea family.

Nature and flavour: Sweet, slightly puckery and moderate.

Constituents: Containing sugar, vitamins B_1, B_2 and C, malic acid and citric acid.

Action: Increasing the formation of body fluids, acting as an antitussive, and beneficial to digestion.

Indications: Chronic malaria, pharyngitis, laryngitis, inner heat of the body, and hotness in urination.

55. Betel nut

The fruit of a plant belonging to the palma family.

Nature and flavour: Warm and pungent.

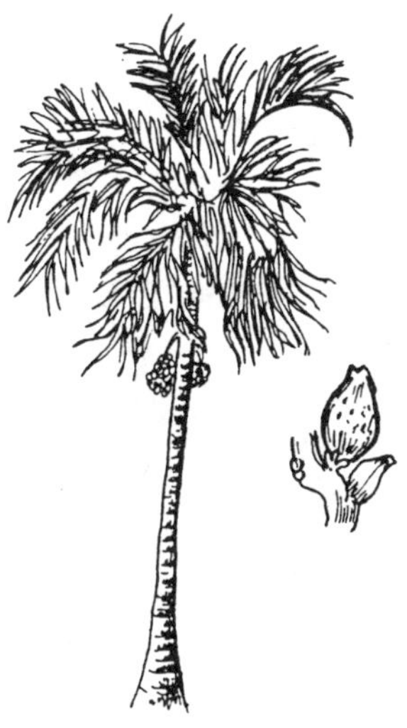

Constituents: Containing much alkaloid, tannate, fat and areca red, with arecaline as its main constituent.

Action: It possesses the action of eliminating abdominal distention, evil-dampness and anthelminthes.

Indications: Clonarchiasis, tapeworm, malaria, influenza. For nephritic edema, make a decoction with betel-nut skin.

56. Cucumber

The fruit of plant belonging to the cucurbitacea family. It can be served raw.

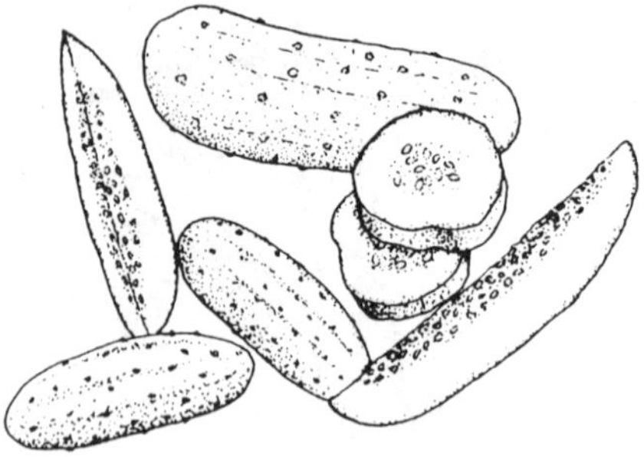

Nature and flavour: Sweet and cold.

Constituents: Containing sugar, protein, vitamin C and volatile oil. Its base is slightly bitter containing cucurbitacin A, B, C, and D.

Action: It clears evil heat, eliminates evil-dampness and has a detoxifying action.

Indications: An ideal remedy for clearing summer heat and eliminating evil dampness during summer days. Also a remedy for boils and carbuncles in summer.

D. Animals

1. Chicken

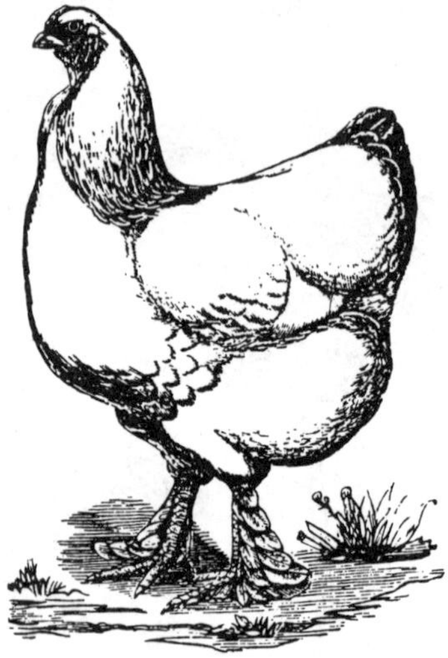

A fowl belonging to the phasianidae family. Almost all its body parts have medical uses. However, chicken flesh, the inner layer of the gizzard and eggs are the most commonly used.

Nature and flavour: Flesh, sweet and warm; and egg, sweet and moderate.

Constituents: Flesh, rich in protein, fat, calcium, phosphorus, iron, and vitamins A, B, C and E; and egg, basically same as those of flesh. In the inner layer of gizzard, there is ventriculin.

Action: Strongly nourishing for all the internal viscera, while the gizzard's inner layer is helpful to digestion. The bile of chicken is good for pertussis.

Indications: General weakness of the body resulting from disease, or postpartum. Functional haemorrhage of uterus and irregular menstruation.

2. Duck

A fowl belonging to the anatidae family.

Nature and flavour: Sweet and cold.

Constituents: Basically the same as those of chicken, with magnesium, potassium and sodium.

Action: General nourishing of weakness.

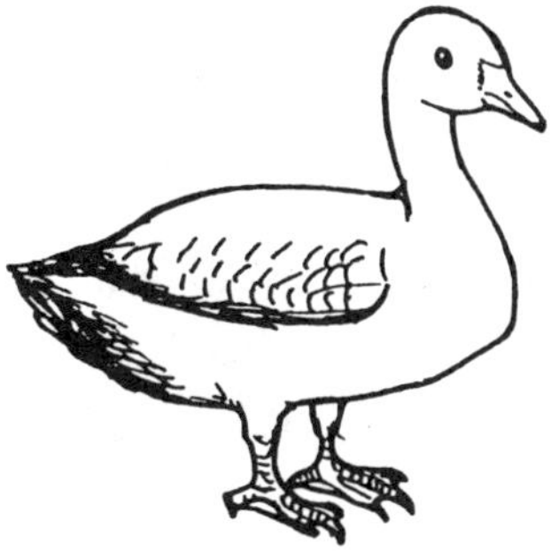

Indications: Weakness, especially yin-deficiency leading to flaming up of evil fire (pathological hyperfunction) neurasthenia, asthma and waist pains in the elderly.

Note: For weakness like hypertension with dizziness, duck is preferable. In TCM, chicken flesh is claimed as wind-type and is not suitable for patients with dizziness due to blood deficiency, while duck flesh is claimed as water-type, so it is preferable for those with deficiency of yin-principle and weakness of the kidney.

3. Sparrow

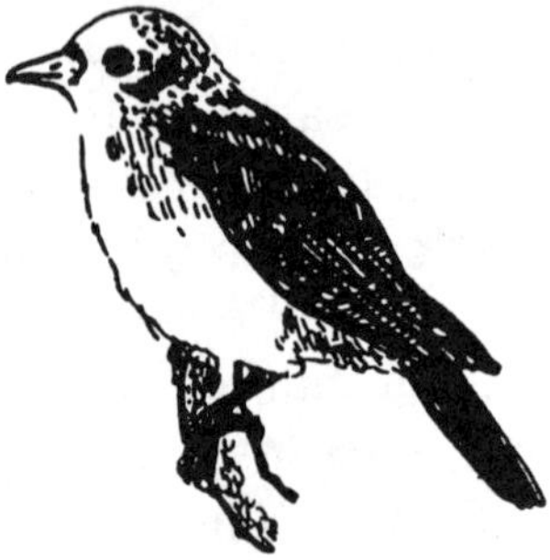

A fowl belonging to the ave family.

Nature and flavour: Sweet and warm.

Constituents: Containing protein, fat, calcium, phosphorus and iron.

Action: Its flesh reinforces sexual activity, warms the waist and knees, and treats profuse metrorrhagia and polyuria due to insufficiency of the kidney.

Indications: Impotence and pertussis.

4. Cormorant

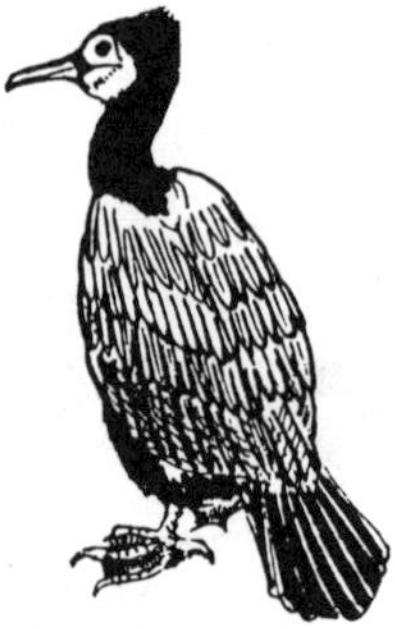

A fowl belonging to the phalacrocoracidae family. Its saliva is also a kind of medicine.

Nature and flavour: Sour and salty.

Constituents: Its flesh is rich in protein.

Action: Diuretic.

Indications: Distension of the abdomen. Its saliva is good for fishbone stuck in the pharynx.

5. Pig

An animal belonging to the suidae family. The commonest domesticated animal in China, with its meat, skin and viscera all used for medical purposes.

Nature and flavour: Flesh, sweet and slightly cold; skin, sweet and cold; bile, bitter and cold; stomach, sweet and warm; and liver, sweet, warm and moderate.

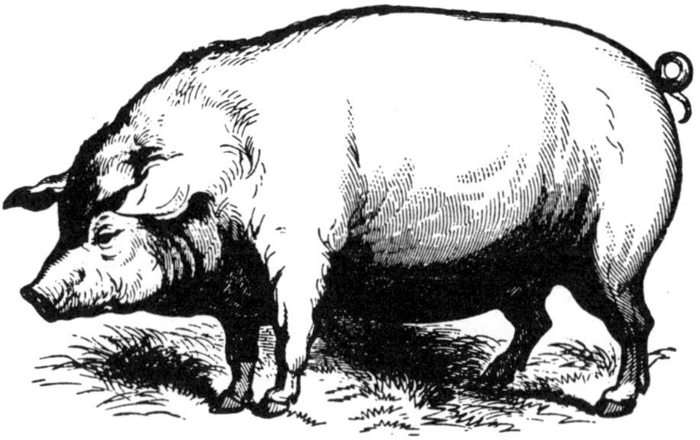

Constituents: Lean flesh is rich in protein; skin, rich in gelatinous protein; liver, rich in iron, protein and vitamin A; bile, bilirubin; and stomach, digestive enzyme.

Action: Flesh, nourishing to weakness; skin, a subsidiary remedy for hemoptysis, nasal bleeding and for regulating menstruation; liver, good for improving eye-sight and as a blood tonic.

Indications: For anaemia and weakness, cook flesh and liver in water with 10 g of angelica sinensis. For dyspepsia, stew stomach with lotus seed and take once daily for several days. For irregular menstruation leading to anaemia, use 200 g of skin simmered until it becomes sticky, then take regularly, eating both skin and soup.

Note: For hypertension and overweight patients, do not take too much pork, especially lard and viscera. Patients with common cold should also avoid such food.

6. Sheep

An animal belonging to the bovida family, with different species such as goat, sheep, wild goat, Mongolian gazelle, etc.

Nature and flavour: Mutton, sweet and hot; and bile, bitter and cold.

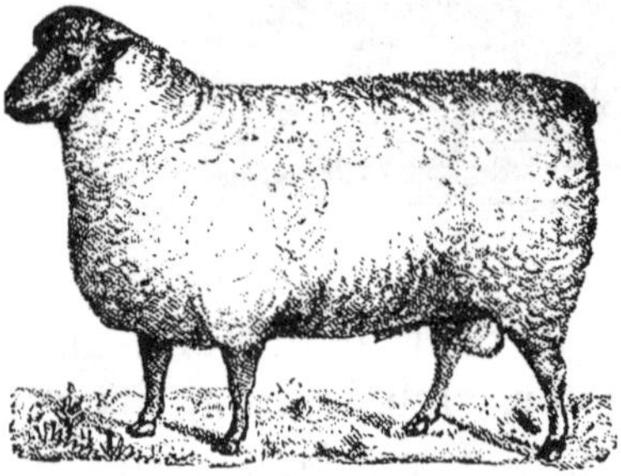

Constituents: Mutton is rich in protein, fat, inorganic salt and vitamins. Its liver is rich in vitamin A.

Action: Mutton is nourishing and warming and is beneficial to weakness and helpful to digestion; and its liver, good for eyesight.

Indications: When stewed with angelica sinensis, it is especially good for postpartum mothers. Its horn is capable of eliminating evil wind and is an antipyretic.

7. Cow

An animal belonging to the bovida family, including buffalo, cow, yak, etc.

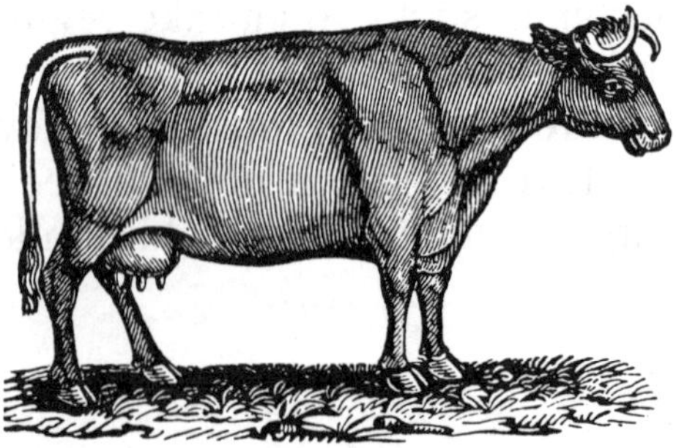

Nature and flavour: Beef, sweet and warm; and horn, bitter and cold.

Constituents: Beef is rich in protein of good

quality, fat, inorganic salt, vitamins and cholesterol. Milk is sweet and cold, and is a very common nutritional food.

Action: Beef is beneficial to the whole body, especially to tendons and bones, eliminating edema. The milk is good for the heart and lungs, stopping thirst. Its horn is an antipyretic in epidemic diseases and is good for hemoptysis and epistaxis.

Indications: Weakness after illness and chronic diarrhoea.

8. Dog

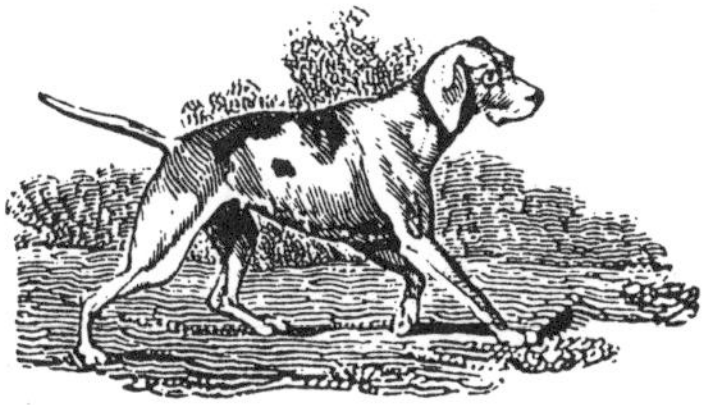

An animal belonging to the caninae family.

Nature and flavour: Salty and hot.

Constituents: Containing purine and carnosine. Also creatine in fresh meat.

Action: Resisting cold and warming the waist and knees. Making one strong.

Indications: Weakness in elderly, chronic malaria.

9. Rabbit

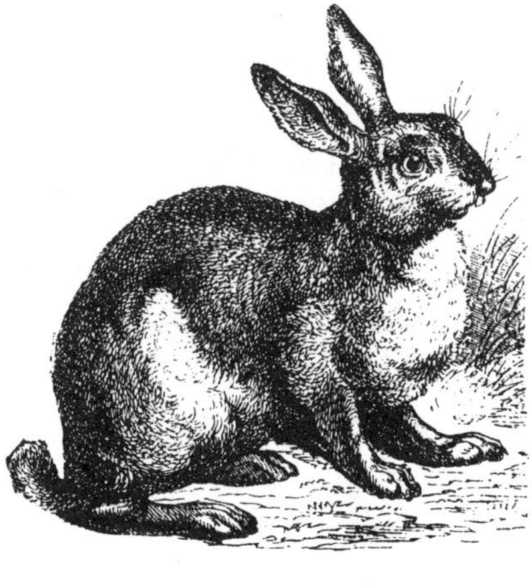

An animal belonging to the eporidae family. Its meat, liver and brain are all used for medicinal purposes.

Nature and flavour: Sweet and cool.

Constituents: Rich in protein. Each 100 g of meat contains 21.2 g of protein, 16 mg of calcium and 2 mg of iron.

Action: Flesh is good for general weakness. The brain possesses oxytocic action. The liver improves eyesight, and relieves night blindness and dizziness.

Indications: Flesh is good for emaciation; liver, for night blindness; and brain, for delivery.

10. Carp

A fish belonging to the cyprinidae family, with different colours, yellow, white and red.

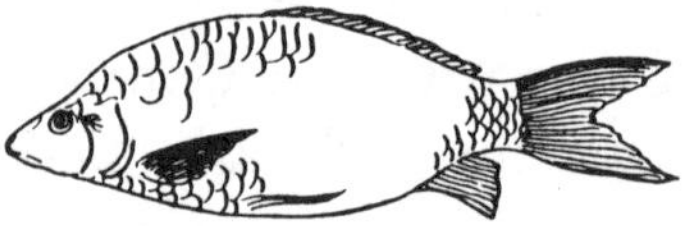

Nature and flavour: Sweet and moderate.

Constituents: Containing protein, fat, calcium, phosphorus, vitamins A and B and nicotinic acid.

Action: Nourishing, benefiting digestion and improving milk secretion and diuretic. A sedative for pregnant women.

Indications: Edema during pregnancy, postpartum shortage of milk secretion, and chronic peptic ulcer.

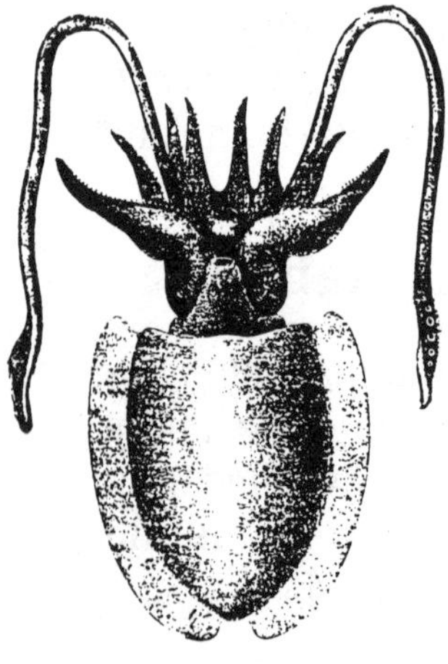

11. Inkfish

A fish belonging to the sepiada family. It has a solitary bone in its interior.

Nature and flavour: Salty and slightly warm.

Constituents: Containing protein, with calcium carbonate in its bone.

Action: Nourishing. The bone is a hemostat, an astringent and an ideal antiacid.

Indications: Gastric and duodenal ulcers, hemoptysis in pulmonary tuberculosis.

12. Snakehead fish

A fish belonging to the mura enesocidae family, black in colour with small scales.

Nature and flavour: Sweet and cold.

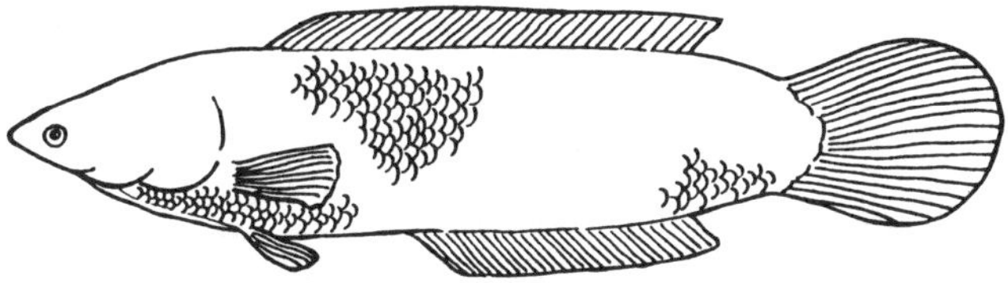

Constituents: Containing protein, fat, calcium, phosphorus, and vitamins A and B.

Action: Benefiting spleen and stomach. Diuretic and eliminating edema.

Indications: Edema, either due to cardiac or kidney diseases.

13. Finless eel

A fish belonging to the branchio sauridae family, yellow in colour, without scales, covered with mucus.

Nature and flavour: Sweet, hot.

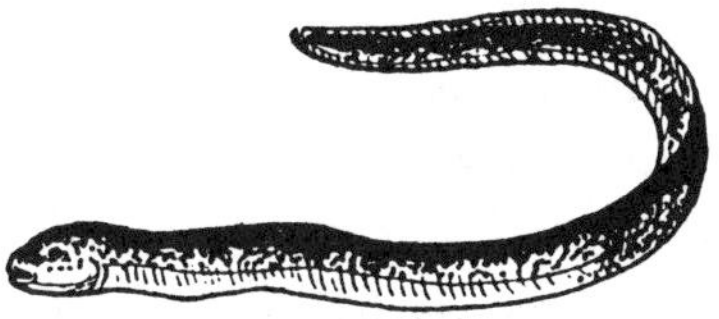

Constituents: Containing protein, fat, inorganic salt and vitamins A and B.

Action: Beneficial to vital energy, nourishing the blood and general deficiency.

Indications: Haemorrhage due to internal haemorrhoid, prolapse of the rectum due to deficiency of vital energy. For facial paralysis and epistaxis, use its blood for local application.

14. Loach

A fish belonging to the cobitidae family.

Nature and flavour: Sweet and moderate.

Constituents: Containing protein, fat, vitamins A, B and B_2, iron, and calcium.

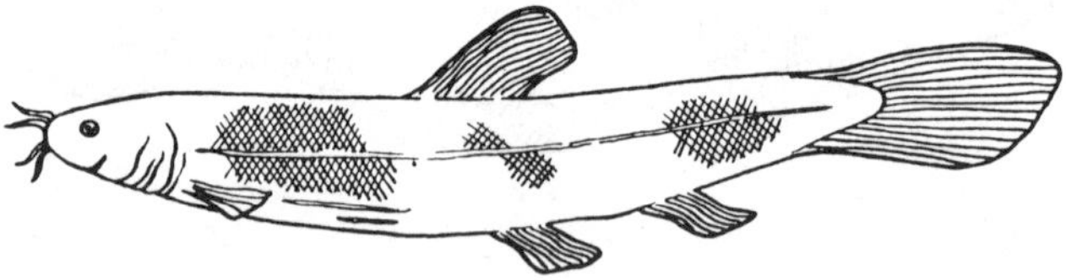

Pharmacology: Its mucilaginous secretion is bacterial inhibiting and anti-inflammatory. In TCM, it is claimed that loach warms the interior of the body and nourishes vital energy.

Indications: Acute and chronic hepatitis, acute cholecystitis. Local application for erysipelas and carbuncles.

15. Tortoise/Turtle

An animal belonging to the testudinidae family. Its abdominal plate is most commonly used for medicinal purposes.

Nature and flavour: Sweet and moderate.

Constituents: Containing protein, fat, vitamins.

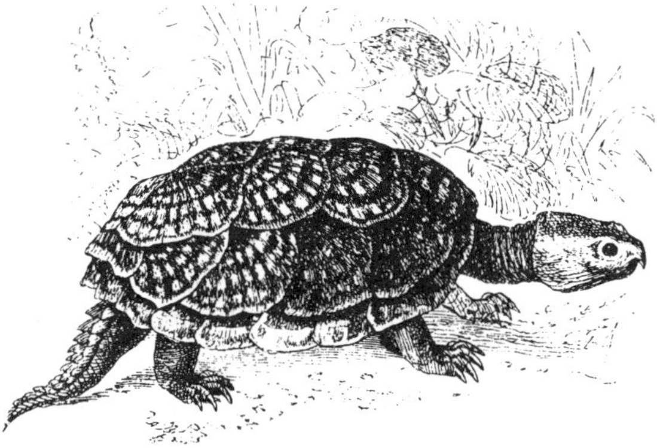

Action: For rheumatism, weakness in the lower extremities, abdominal lumps and chronic malaria.

Indications: Chronic dyspepsia in children, emaciation, chronic malaria and tuberculosis.

16. Soft shell turtle

An animal belonging to the trionychidae family. The whole body, especially its abdominal plate, is used for medicinal purposes.

Nature and flavour: Salty and moderate.

Constituents: Containing gelatinous protein, fat, kerain, sugar, inorganic salt, and vitamins A, B, B_2 and D.

Action: Good for tuberculous fever, eliminating lumps in abdomen in chronic malaria. Its blood nourishes the

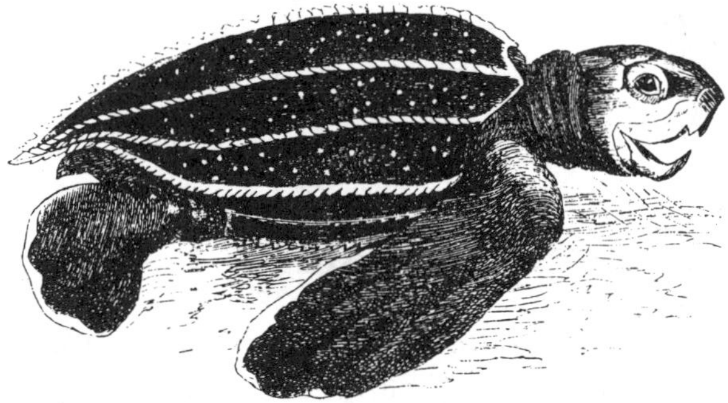

yin-principle (vital essence of the body) and reduces fever.

Indications: Chronic malaria, afternoon fever in tuberculosis. The turtle head baked and ground into powder is applied for prolapse of the rectum and uterus.

17. Pangolin

The scales are used for medicinal purposes.

Nature and flavour: Salty and cool.

Constituents: The scales contain animal gelatin, calcium phosphate and protein.

Action: Eliminating swelling and lumps, clearing the channels, facilitating pus drainage, milk secretion and menstruation.

Indications: For shortage of milk secretion, boils before pus formation and as a hemostat applied locally.

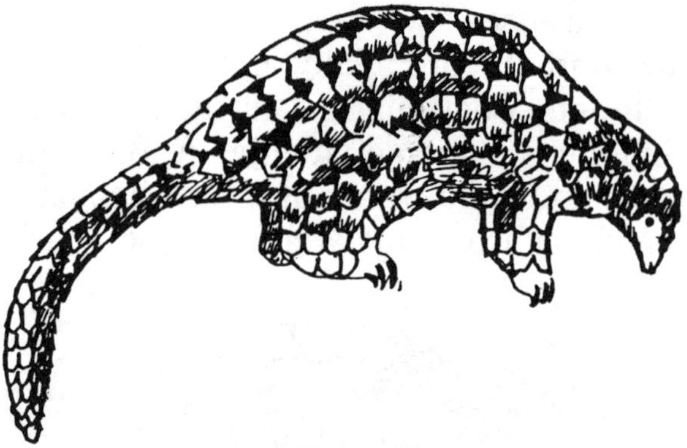

18. Freshwater clam

A shellfish belonging to the anodontae family.

Nature and flavour: Salty and cold.

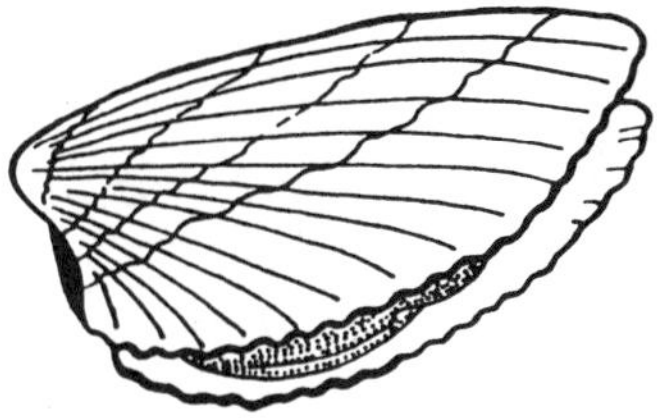

Constituents: Protein, fat, sugar, calcium, vitamins A, B_1 and B_2. Its shell and pearl contain large amounts of calcium carbonate and magnesium carbonate.

Action: Stopping thirst, eliminating fever and detoxifying. The nacre is used as a remedy for dizziness and excess of liver function.

Indications: Thirst, red eyes due to deficient vital essence. Local application for sore throat, red eyes and nebula.

19. River snail

A shellfish belonging to the paludinae family.

Nature and flavour: Sweet and cold.

Constituents: Containing protein, inorganic salt, vitamins A, B_1, B_2 and D.

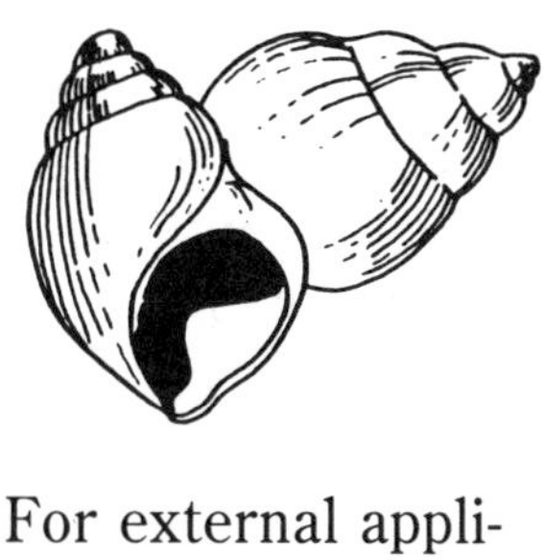

Action: Beneficial to urination and defecation. Relieving summer heat and is antipyretic.

Indications: For jaundice due to evil heat and dampness, rickets in children, diabetes with polyuria. For external application in edema and anal prolapse.

20. Oyster

A shellfish belonging to the ostreidae family. Both the shell and the flesh are used for medicinal purposes.

Nature and flavour: Salty and slightly cold.

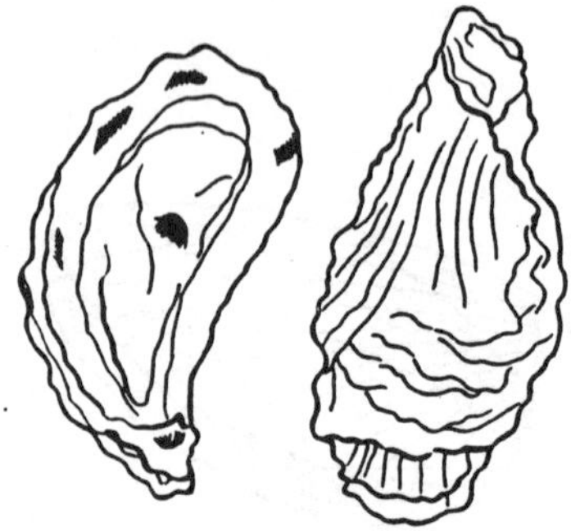

Constituents: The flesh contains sugar, lipoid, vitamins, and fucose; and its shell, calcium carbonate, magnesium, aluminium and ferrous oxide.

Action: An excellent nutrient for deficiency of vital essence. Its shell is a sedative and antiacid.

Indications: Tuberculous lymphadenitis and weakness. Night sweating, insomnia, palpitation and emission due to neuraasthenia can be cured by its shell.

21. Jellyfish

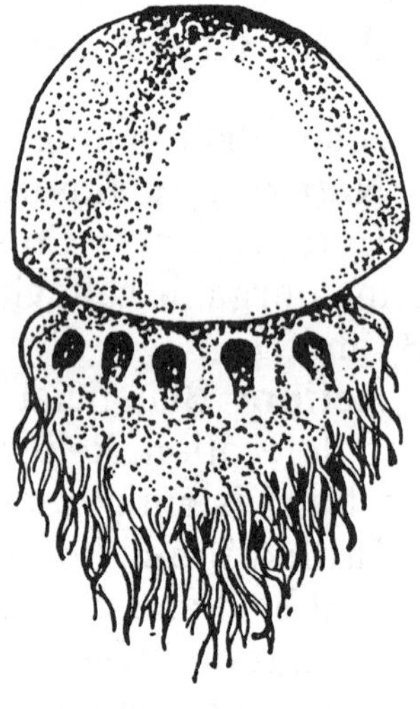

Belonging to the rhopilemada family.

Nature and flavour: Salty and warm.

Constituents: Containing protein, fat, sugar, inorganic salt and vitamins A and B.

Pharmacology: In animal experiments, it has been shown to lower blood pressure. In TCM, it is claimed that it softens hard masses, eliminates sputum and cures wind and heat in children.

Indications: Hypertension, acute bronchitis with yellow and sticky sputum.

E. Processed Food and Flavourings

1. Salt

There are different kinds of salt produced from sea, well and lake water, as well as rock salt.

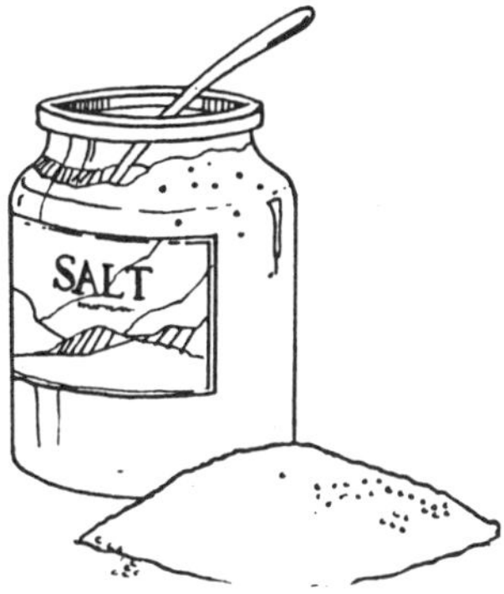

Nature and flavour: Salty and cold.

Constituents: Mainly sodium chloride. There are more impurities in sea water salt, such as considerate amount of iodine, potassium chloride, magnesium sulphate, calcium sulphate, etc.

Action: Regulating the spleen-stomach functions, detoxifying food poisoning.

Indications: For food poisoning, rinsing the stomach with saline water to induce vomiting. Putting hot salt on the navel and then using moxibustion on top is good for stopping anuria and hernia pains.

2. Alcoholic drinks

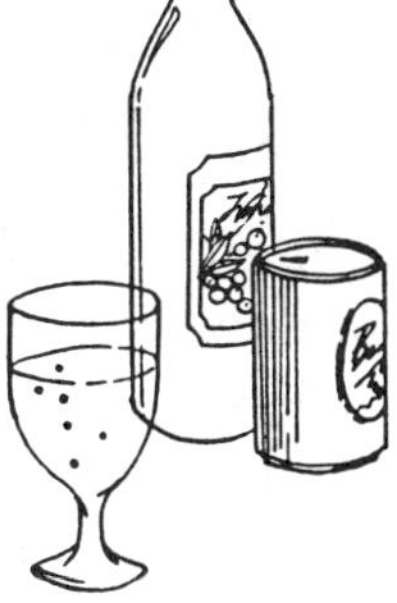

There are a great variety of alcoholic drinks used, including Chinese white liquor, wine, rice wine, etc.

Nature and flavour: Sweet, pungent, warm or hot.

Constituents: Mainly alcohol in different concentrations from 10-70 percent.

Action: Invigorating blood circulation resulting in the promotion of the therapeutic effect of medicines and eliminating evil-wind. Analgesic action.

Indications: Rheumatism of joints and soft tissues, neuralgia. Also for wounds when external massage is applied. The therapeutic action of some drugs is reinforced when soaked in alcohol.

3. Vinegar

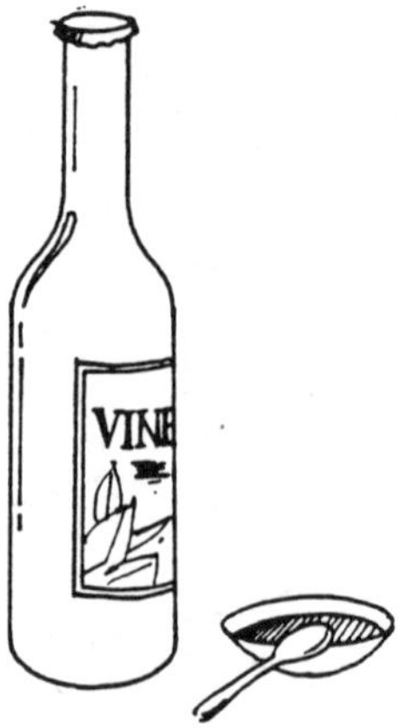

Commonly produced by fermentation of grains, hence the name rice vinegar. There are different kinds of vinegar due to the different processing methods and original materials used.

Nature and flavour: Sour and warm.

Constituents: Mainly acetic acid and some vitamins B_1 and B_2.

Action: Antiseptic and relieving swelling. Refreshing the brain when its vapour is inhaled.

Indications: Acute infectious hepatitis. Ascaris in the digestive tracts, anaphylactia of digestive tract due to animal protein.

4. Processed soybean

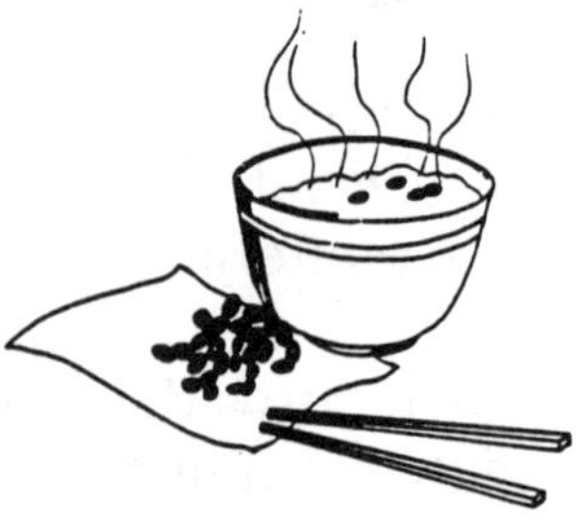

Made by the fermentation of boiled black beans.

Nature and flavour: Bitter and cold.

Constituents: Protein and vitamins B_1 and B_2.

Action: Antipyretic, and diaphretic to relieve the exterior symptom complex. Detoxifying and promoting eruption of rash in measles.

Indications: Early stages of the common cold when there is fever, headache with no sweating or little sweating. Also effective for night sweating and dysentery.

5. Scorched rice crust

The yellow crust formed at the bottom of the pan when cooking rice.

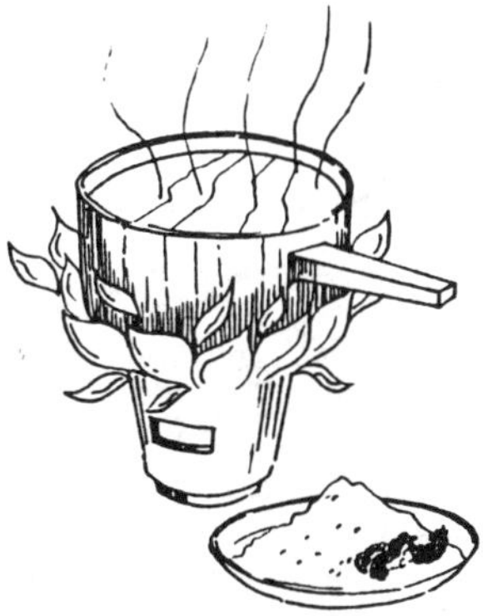

Nature and flavour: Sweet, moderate, and slightly warm.

Constituents: Mainly starch.

Action: Good for digestion, and promoting the secretion of digestive fluids.

Indications: Dyspepsia due to irregular eating and drinking, loss of appetite, chronic gastro-enteritis.

6. Sugar

Made from sugar cane or beet. There are different kinds of sugar including brown, white and rock sugar.

Nature and flavour: Brown sugar, sweet and warm; and rock sugar, sweet and moderate.

Constituents: Mainly sucrose. There is also chlorophyll, xanthophyll, carrotene and inorganic salt in brown sugar.

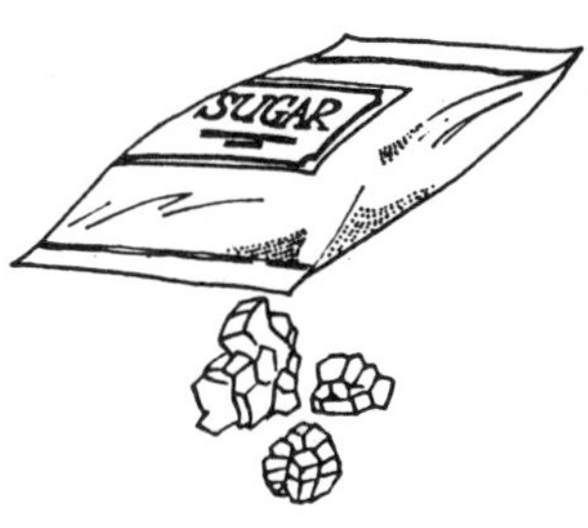

Action: Benefiting the spleen, vital energy circulation and good for digestion. In addition it relieves pain, promotes blood circulation and removes stagnation.

Indications: Brown sugar is administered for women's abdominal pains due to cold attack during menstruation and weakness after delivery. White sugar is good for the lungs. Coupled with other drugs, it is good for coughing.

7. Honey

Made by honey bees, which are domesticated. Wild bee honey is also occasionally used.

Nature and flavour: Sweet and moderate.

Constituents: The contents are very complicated. Apart from glucose, fructose and mallose, there is dextrin, protein, iron, calcium, phosphorus, potassium, manganese, sodium, copper, wax, pigments, natural flavouring, malic acid, lactic acid, formic acid, oxidase, transformase and vitamins B_1, B_2, B_6, D and E.

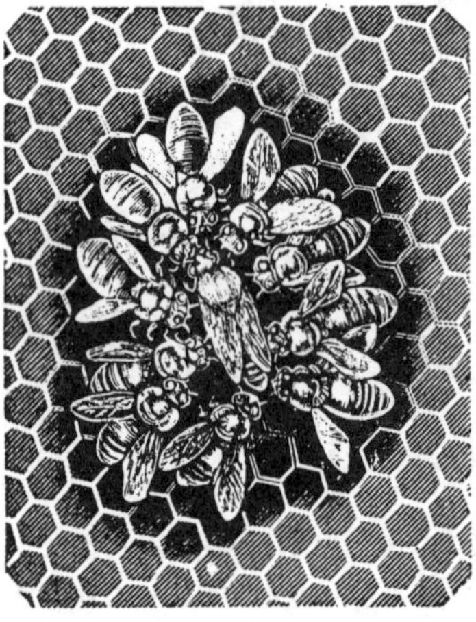

Action: Nourishing the vital energy, benefiting digestion, and regulating the spleen-stomach function. Easing all the internal viscera, detoxification. Moistening the intestines, lowering blood pressure and preventing arterio sclerosis. High nutritional value.

Indications: Hypertension, peptic ulcer, habitual constipation, bronchitis, neurasthenia and general weakness after severe illness.

Appendix 1

Manifestations of Cold, Heat, Deficiency and Excess in TCM*

Manifestations		
High fever, thirst, low voice, constipation, yellow coating on the tongue, red tongue, swift and forceful pulse, sore throat, deep coloured urine, and flushed face.	Heat due to excess	Heat syndrome
Low fever, not thirst, afternoon fever, fatigue, emaciation, scarlet tongue without coating, minute and rapid pulse, and general weakness.	Heat due to deficiency	
Cold extremities, abdominal pains, constipation, sunken and string-like pulse, and white coating on the tongue.	Cold due to excess	Cold syndrome
Loss of appetite, profuse saliva secretion, shortness of breath, diarrhoea with undigested food, pale tongue with white coating, minute and and weak pulse.	Cold due to deficiency	

*Traditional Chinese Medicine

Appendix 2

Manifestations of Excess and Deficiency in Blood and Vital Energy (Qi)

Excess syndrome	*Deficiency syndrome*	
Pallor, lassitude, fatigue and weakness, shortness of breath when moving, dizziness, sweating, and diarrhoea. Sometimes prolapses of anus or uterus.	Accumulation and obstruction of phlegm,. chest and abdominal distention, vomiting with gastric acid, constipation (clinically termed stagnation of vital energy, and excess syndrome of viscera)	Vital energy (qi, yang)
Paleness in face, lips, tongue and nails, numbness and spasm of extremities, nausea, dizziness, palpitation, restlessness, insomnia, night sweating, afternoon fever, hotness in palms and soles.	Abdominal pains during menstruation or postpartum period, tenderness in abdomen. Local blood stagnation and pain after fall (clinically termed blood stagnation)	Blood (yin)

Note: Those patients with qi or yang deficiency should take diets of moderate and warm nature; those with blood or yin deficiency, sweet diets of cold, and cool nature

Appendix 3

Nature of Everyday Food: **Food Moderate in Nature**

Plants: auricularia-auricula judae, spinach

Roots and Stems: sweet potato, taro, potato, Chinese yam

Flowers, Seeds, Gourds and Fruits: sesame, whole wheat, rice, maize, red bean, hyacinth bean, cowpea, black bean, peanut, pumpkin, bottle gourd, lotus seed, black plum, sunflower seed, guava, Chinese date, loquat, water chestnut, gorgon fruit, fruit of Chinese wolfberry, carambola, fruit of white mulberry, lily, chrysanthemum, tomato, gingko

Animals: carp, inkfish, crucian carp, rabbit's meat, pork, egg, milk, loach, tortoise, soft shell turtle

Processed Food and Flavourings: rock sugar, cane sugar, honey

Appendix 4

Nature of Everyday Food: **Food Cold or Cool in Nature**

Plants: peppermint, artemisia, Xianggu mushroom, kelp, seaweed, purslane, laver, spinach, water bamboo, eggplant, celery, cabbage, tremella, cogongrass rhizome

Flowers, Seeds, Gourds and Fruits: husked sorghum, fruit of Job's tear, bean curd, day lily, green bean, soybean, sword bean, gingko, water-melon, pear, lotus root, water chestnut, banana, persimmon, white gourd, cucumber, bitter gourd, guava

Animals: pangolin, clam, fresh-water snail, frog, duck, oyster, snakehead fish

Processed Food and Flavourings: tea, salt, processed bean

Appendix 5

Nature of Everyday Food: **Food Warm or Hot in Nature**

Plants: chive, shallot, onion, garlic, coriander, cinnamon

Roots and Stems: tuber of multiflower knotweed, turnip, carrot

Flowers, Seeds, Gourds and Fruits: fresh wheat, flour, wheat flour, palm starch grain, chestnut, barley, hyacinth bean, broad bean , almond, pomegranate, lichee, longan, areca nut, olive, hawthorn, pepper, Chinese prickly ash, tangerine, orange, chilli, clove, sweet scented osmanthus

Animals: finless eel, chicken, sparrow, pig's liver, dog's meat, mutton, beef, sheep's kidney, sheep's milk, inkfish, snake's meat, jelly fish, sea cucumber

Processed Food and Flavourings: scorched rice crust, coffee, vinegar, wine, brown sugar

Appendix 6

Glossary of Common Medicinal Foods

Acanthaceous indigo tuber 靛（有棘的）
Acanthopanax root bark 三加皮
Alcoholic drinks 酒精
Alfal'fa 紫花苜蓿
Almond 杏仁
Alum 明礬
Angelica sinensis 当归
Aniseed 洋茴香
Apricot 杏仁
Astragali 黄蓍
Atractylodes root 苍术，白术
Auricularia auricula-judae 木耳
Balsam pear 梨
Bamboo 竹
Banana 香蕉
Barley 大麦，薏米
Bean 豆
Bean curd 豆腐
Betel nut 槟榔
Bidentate achyranthes root 牛膝根（双牙的）
Bitter gourd 苦瓜
Black bean 黑豆
Black pepper corn 黑胡椒
Black soya bean 黑豆
Brown sugar 黄砂糖
Calabash 葫芦
Cane sugar 蔗糖
Capillary artemisia 茵陈蒿

Carp 鲤鱼
Carrot 胡萝卜
Celery 芹菜
Chestnut 栗
Chicken 鸡
Chilli 辣椒
Chinese caterpillar fungus 冬虫草
Chinese date 枣
Chinese dodder seed 菟丝子
Chinese sorghum 高粱
Chinese trichosanthes 王瓜，瓜蒌
Chinese yam 山药
Chives 虾夷葱
Chrysanthemum 菊花
Cinnamon 桂皮
Cinnamon cassia bark 肉桂
Clove 丁香，珠芽
Codonopsis pilosula root 党参
Cogongrass root 白茅根
Coriander 香菜
Cormorant 鹈鹕
Cow 牛
Cowpea 豇豆
Crucian carp 醋鱼
Crystal sugar 碎冰糖
Cucumber 小黄瓜
Date 枣
Deer antler 鹿角
Dog 狗
Dried bean skin 豆皮干
Dried longan pulp 干桂圆肉，干龙眼肉
Duck 鸭
Eel 河鳗
Egg 蛋
Eggplant 茄子
Fennel 茴香
Fennel fruit 茴香果
Finless eel 鳗

Fish-head 鱼头
Flour 面粉
Freshwater clam 鲜蚶子
Fructus amomi 砂仁
Fructus psoraleae 补骨脂
Gall-bladder 胆囊
Garlic 大蒜
Gastrodia 天麻
Gastrodia tuber 天麻
Ginger 姜
Gingko 银杏
Gizzard 肫肝
Glutinous rice 糯米
Grape 葡萄
Green bean 绿豆
Green tea 青茶
Guava 番石榴
Hawthorn 山楂
Hen's intestines 鸡肠
Herba cistanchis 肉蓯蓉
Honey 蜜糖
Horse radish 马萝卜
Hyacinth flower 扁花
Inkfish 墨鱼
Jellyfish 海蜇
Job's tear 薏苡仁
Kelp 海草，海带
Kumquat 金橘
Laver 紫菜
Lichee 荔枝
Licorice root 草果，甘草
Lily 百合花
Liquor 酒
Liver 肝
Loquat 枇杷
Lotus root 莲藕
Lotus seed 莲子
Maize 玉米

Mare's milk 马奶
Milk vetch 野豌豆奶，沙苑
Mulberry 桑
Mung bean 绿豆
Mustard 芥菜
Mutton 羊肉
Noodles 面条
Nuts 豆
Olive 橄榄
Onion 洋葱
Orange 橙
Orange peel 陈皮
Osmanthus flower 桂花
Oyster 蚝
Pangolin 穿山甲
Pangolin scales 穿山甲鳞
Papaya 木瓜
Peanut 花生
Peanut skin 花生皮
Pear 梨
Peppermint 薄荷
Pericarpium zanthoxyli 花椒
Persimmon 柿子
Pig 猪
Pig's bone 猪骨
Pig's brain 猪脑
Pig's gall-bladder 猪胆囊
Pig's kidney 猪腰
Pig's liver 猪肝
Pig's lung 猪肺
Pig's pancreas 猪胰
Pig's skin 猪皮
Pig's stomach 猪肚
Pig's trotters 猪脚
Plantain 车前草
Plum 李子，梅子
Polygonum multiflorum 何首乌
Pomegranate 石榴

Pomegranate peel 石榴皮
Poria 茯苓
Pork 猪肉
Porridge 粥
Pumpkin 南瓜
Purslane 马齿苋
Rabbit 兔
Rapeseed 油菜子
Red beans 红豆
Rhizoma atractylodis 苍术
Rhizoma drynariae 骨碎补
Rice 米
Rice crust 饭焦，锅巴
Rice stem 米梗
Rice wine 米酒
Rice-paper plant 通草
River snail 河蜗牛，河响螺
Rock candy 冰糖
Saffron 番红花
Salt 盐
Scallion 葱
Scorched rice crust 锅巴，饭焦
Sea cucumber 海参
Seaweed 海草
Sesame oil 芝麻油
Sheep 羊
Sheep's bone 羊骨
Sheep's kidney 羊腰
Silver carp 银鲤鱼
Smilax glabra 土茯苓
Snail 蜗牛
Snakehead fish 蛇头鱼
Soft shell turtle 软壳甲，水鱼
Soy sauce 酱油
Soybeans 黄豆
Sparrow 麻雀
Spices 香料
Spinach 菠菜

Starch 浆
Sugar 糖
Sunflower disc 向日葵子
Sweet potato 番薯
Sword beans 剑豆
Tangerine peel 蜜橘皮
Taro 芋头
Tea 茶
Tomato 番茄
Tortoise/turtle 龟/甲鱼，水鱼
Turnip 白萝卜
Vermicelli 通心面条，粉丝，干米粉
Vinegar 醋
Viscera 内脏
Walnut 胡桃
Water chestnut 马蹄，荸荠
Water melon 西瓜
Wheat 小麦
Wheat bran 糠
White gourd 白瓜
White melon 白瓜
White pepper corn 白胡椒
White sugar 白糖
Wild duck 蚬鸭
Wild jujube seed 酸枣仁
Wolfberry seed 枸杞子

CHINESE CULTURE SERIES

150x210mm, fully illustrated

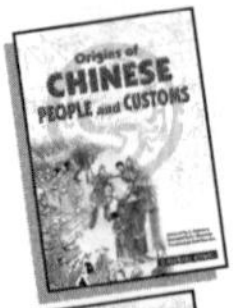

ORIGINS OF CHINESE PEOPLE AND CUSTOMS
Explores the beginnings of the Chinese people, origins of Chinese names, Chinese zodiac signs, the afterlife, social etiquette and more!

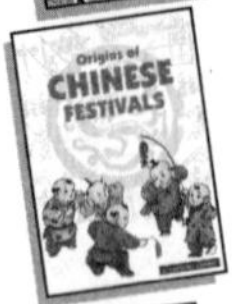

ORIGINS OF CHINESE FESTIVALS
Stories about Lunar New Year, Chinese Valentine's Day, Qing Ming, Dragon Boat, Zhong Yuan, Mid-Autumn Festivals and more.

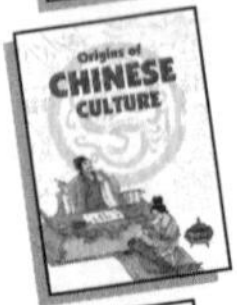

ORIGINS OF CHINESE CULTURE
Previously **'ORIGINS OF CHINESE MUSIC AND ART'**
Interesting facts about the "Four Treasures of the Study": the brush, ink, paper and inkstone, which form the cornerstone of Chinese culture.

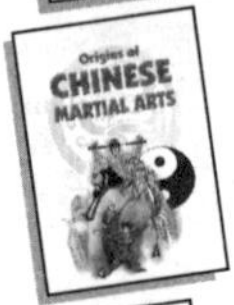

ORIGINS OF CHINESE MARTIAL ARTS
Traces the origins of the *gongfu* of Shaolin and Wudang warriors and their philosophy and chivalry code.

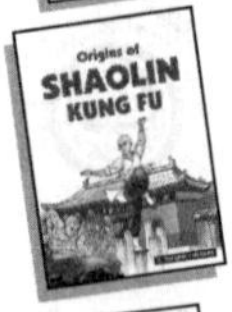

ORIGINS OF SHAOLIN KUNG FU
An entertaining read for all budding martial arts enthusiasts and all who want to explore the wonders of Shaolin Kung Fu!

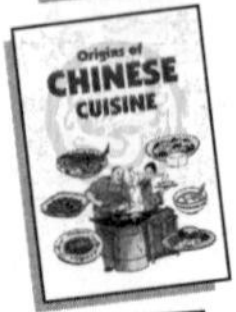

ORIGINS OF CHINESE CUISINE
Showcases famous and best-relished dishes, including Peking Roast Duck and Buddha Jumps Over the Wall, and the stories behind them.

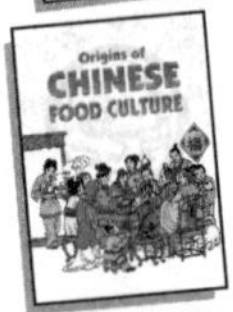

ORIGINS OF CHINESE FOOD CULTURE
Covers the origins, history, customs, and the art and science of Chinese food culture, including the 18 methods of cooking.

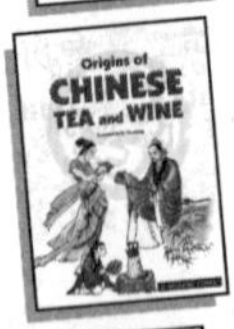

ORIGINS OF CHINESE TEA AND WINE
Tea and wine have a long history in China. In fact, both have become firmly entrenched in the culture and customs of the Chinese people.

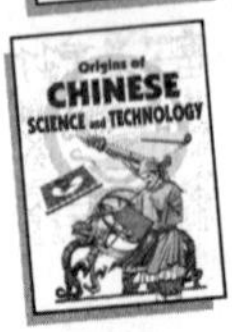

ORIGINS OF CHINESE SCIENCE & TECHNOLOGY
Covers great inventions by the Chinese: the compass, paper-making, gunpowder and printing. Also explores Chinese expertise in the fields of geography, mathematics, agriculture and astronomy.

ESSENCE OF TRADITIONAL CHINESE MEDICINE
Compiled by **Asiapac Editorial**, illustrated by **Fu Chunjiang**
150x210mm, 192pp, ISBN 981-229-364-7

The art of Chinese medicine has been in existence for thousands of years. Its unique methods of diagnosis and treatment are known throughout the world. Its mystique lies in its apparent simplicity. Without the need for complicated equipment and apparatus, it is often able to diagnose and treat patients with surprising results.

The enormous scope of Chinese medicine can be intimidating. This book attempts to put across its fundamental concepts in everyday language that anyone can understand. Interesting stories about its history have also been included to enliven the reader's introduction to the wondrous world of Chinese medicine, with its vast and rich treasure trove of information.

- The Four Diagnoses — Observation, Olfaction, Interrogation and Pulse-taking
- Chinese medicines, acupuncture and moxibustion, diet therapy, *qigong*...
- Famous Physicians — Bian Que, Hua Tuo, Zhang Zhongjing, Sun Simiao, Zhu Danxi, Li Shizhen
- Yin-yang and the five elements; eight principal syndromes
- Bodily fluids, vital energy, blood, meridians and collaterals

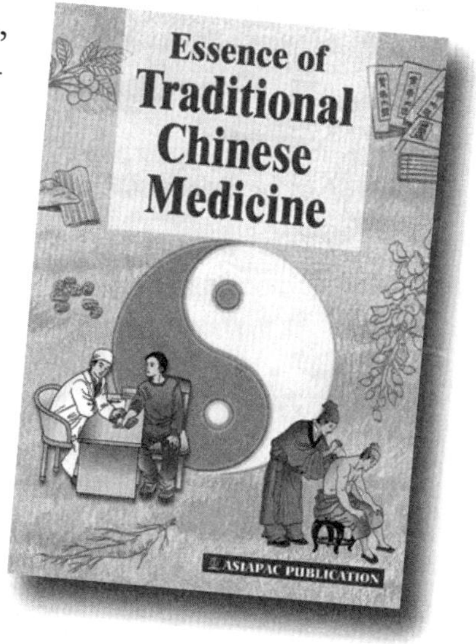

中医饮食疗法

作者 ：蔡景峰

亚太图书有限公司出版